# PRAISE FOR TORN

"*Torn* offers up the finest imaginable gift for today's moms, no matter whether you work or stay at home: the comforting truth that we all juggle life and kids as best we can, and that moms ride this nutty 'mommy wars' roller coaster together. Moms will laugh, cry, identify – and feel an invaluable sense of validation that modern motherhood is more challenging, and more joyful, than anyone ever told us."

– Leslie Morgan Steiner, author of *Mommy Wars* and *New York Times* Bestseller *Crazy Love*

"A fascinating look at Mothering 2.0. In *Torn*, a new generation of mothers explores the delicate balancing act of work and family life with intelligence, wit, and candor."

– Willow Bay, Senior Editor, *The Huffington Post,* and Special Correspondent, Bloomberg Television

"*Torn* is a heartfelt look at how a generation of mothers is trying to forge its own identity while honoring the legacy of '60s and '70s feminism. Sometimes freedom can be its own trap, and this book illustrates that principle beautifully."

– Neal Pollack, columnist for *Vanity Fair* and author of *Alternadad* and *Stretch*

"Suffice it to say that I started reading the book in the subway and missed my stop! These little essays, often poignant, capture where American mothers find themselves today."

– Joan C. Williams, Distinguished Professor of Law & Founder/ Director of the Center for Work-Life Law, University of California, Hastings College of the Law

"With *Torn*, Samantha Walravens offers a diverse collection of voices making a valuable contribution to our ongoing discussion about trying to maintain a career while raising a family. These writers are sometimes rueful and sometimes quite raw, but always compellingly honest. They insist we set aside guilt and judgment and instead listen to their truths – complicated and difficult as they are – in the hope that someday our children will feel less torn."

– Caroline Grant, Editor-in-Chief, LiteraryMama.com and co-editor, *Mama, PhD: Women Write About Motherhood and Academic Life*

"A tender, humorous, and sometimes heartbreaking collection of experiences as unique as the women who lived them. For those of us who were guided, and often defined, by the women's movement, these stories resonate in a way that is both sustaining and essential."

– Victoria Zackheim, Editor, *He Said What? Women Write About Moments When Everything Changed*

"Finally, a reality-based look at life, love and motherhood *for* real women *from* real women. No quick fixes or fantasy escapes here. Just good, old-fashioned, in-the-trenches camaraderie that lets you know you are not alone and that the fight is worth it. Really!"

– Allison Glock, author of the award-winning memoir *Beauty Before Comfort* and mother of two girls she still hugs in public

"*Torn* speaks a bold, discomfiting truth: there is no easy solution when it comes to balancing career and parenting. These unflinchingly honest stories reveal the unusually high stakes of women's choices about work and family – for their marriage, their children, their career, their financial life, and especially for their own identity. This book is a vital contribution to the conversation about the value of domestic life and the hidden costs of work for women and their families. Offering neither easy solutions nor judgment, its hope lies in its willingness to fully engage the messy realities that so many women face every day."

– Lisa Harper, author of *A Double Life, Discovering Motherhood* (Winner of the 2010 River Teeth Literary Nonfiction Award)

"In a culture that obsesses over every conceivable determinant of woman's identity – from physical appearance to marital status, from mothering skills to career potential – the real women behind the societal images often get lost. Finally, forty-seven successful, well-educated women have taken on the challenging task of telling it like it is, relaying their stories of how they manage (or not) to balance career and motherhood, professional life with the demands of family. These essays promise to entertain and answer the question asked by every generation of women: is it possible to do it all?"

– Karen Carrera, former Deputy City Attorney, San Francisco, and board member, Equal Rights Advocates

"Sharp, poignant and sometimes funny stories about some very unfunny issues that mothers grapple with daily. If you have a mother, are a mother or know a mother, read this book."

– Katherine Clifford, Founder of Youronramp.com

"As a therapist who sees many women 'torn' between the conflicting demands of motherhood, marriage and career, I believe that the deep empathy and understanding created by these remarkably honest and moving personal testimonies makes this book a 'must read' both for women struggling to create work-life balance and for men trying to understand the plight of the women in their lives."

– Geraldine Alpert, PhD, Licensed Clinical Psychotherapist and Associate Clinical Professor of Psychiatry, University of California Medical School, San Francisco

# TORN

# TORN

## TRUE STORIES OF KIDS, CAREER & THE CONFLICT OF MODERN MOTHERHOOD

EDITED BY

SAMANTHA PARENT WALRAVENS

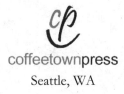

coffeetownpress

Seattle, WA

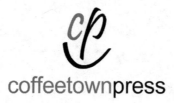

coffeetownpress

Coffeetown Press
PO Box 70515
Seattle, WA 98127

For more information contact: www.coffeetownpress.com

Cover illustration by Kristie Langone, www.2FacedDesign.com
Cover design by Sabrina Sun

TORN: TRUE STORIES OF KIDS, CAREER & THE
CONFLICT OF MODERN MOTHERHOOD
Copyright © 2011 by Samantha Parent Walravens

ISBN: 978-1-60381-097-5 (Trade Paperback)
Library of Congress Control Number: 2011923303
10 9 8 7 6 5 4 3 2

Printed in the United States of America

To Matthew, Zachary, Colette and Gigi,
who gave me the inspiration to write this book.

# ACKNOWLEDGMENTS

This book would not be possible without the efforts of the women who were brave enough to write candidly about their lives and the difficult choices that women today must make when it comes to raising kids and pursuing careers. A heartfelt thank you goes out to my husband, Patrick, for supporting me throughout the writing process and giving me valuable feedback on the manuscript; to my friend, Karen, who has struggled, laughed and cried beside me during this impossible journey of motherhood; to my beloved friend and guardian angel, Crissy, who taught me to pursue my dreams despite the obstacles life puts in front of you; and to all the Princeton alumni who helped bring this book to fruition. I cannot thank you enough.

# CONTENTS

# INTRODUCTION

*I've yet to be on a campus where most women weren't worrying about some aspect of combining marriage, children, and a career. I've yet to find one where many men were worrying about the same thing.*

– Gloria Steinem

The pressure caught up to me one day, back when I was working crazy hours at a Silicon Valley Internet startup. It was during the dot-com bubble of the 1990s, when employees were selling their souls to their employers for the sake of stock options that promised a small fortune, if not an early retirement. After a horrific two-hour commute home along a backed-up freeway, I found myself in the kitchen, screaming at my husband to make his own dinner while throwing a box of breakfast cereal on the table in front of our two-year-old son. They looked at me, bewildered. My inner good girl, who thought she could do it all, had snapped.

Women of my generation – those who came of age in the 1970s and '80s – made a critical error. We interpreted the Women's Movement, which freed us from domestic bondage and opened the doors to economic opportunity, as a mandate to achieve the impossible: the happy marriage, the lovely home, the right wardrobe, the Norman Rockwell holidays, the satisfying career, the accomplished children, and whatever else friends and neighbors were claiming as the "must have" of the moment. Motherhood? Sure, we could do that in our down time, but it was not something we aspired to.

While much of the change that has happened over the past few decades has benefited women enormously, it has come with a cost.

In trying to have it all, women today have pushed themselves to the limit. They feel overworked and under-appreciated. Moreover, they feel *torn*: torn between the conflicting demands of career and family; torn between the desire to achieve and the expectation to selflessly serve those around them. Whether they work, stay at home, or do both, they are judged for not living up to their potential: those who focus on career are criticized for not fulfilling the role of a traditional mother; those who stay home to raise children are criticized for "opting out" and not pursuing their professional goals; those who juggle part-time work and motherhood are seen as doing a mediocre job in both areas.

My moment of reckoning had come. I realized at that moment, box of Cheerios in hand, that despite my best efforts to be a good mother, wife, and worker, I simply could not do it all. I felt duped. Nobody had ever told me that I would have to make a choice: that ambition and motherhood were mutually exclusive goals.

I downshifted to part-time, which curtailed my hopes for promotion and career advancement but gave me more time at home with my son. With the birth of my second child, I made the difficult decision to quit my job altogether. Financially, we could make it on one salary. Emotionally, my pride and self-confidence were squashed to the ground. I had been a go-getter, an achiever, a Princeton Phi Beta Kappa grad. Now I was a "stay-at-home" mom to two little boys. I didn't need a diploma to do this job.

True, my decision to quit was a dilemma of the privileged. The vast majority of American women simply don't have the choice to stay home and raise their kids. But quitting my job to be a stay-at-home mom is not what I had hoped for or expected of myself; nor did I find the experience of changing dirty diapers and breast feeding every two hours fulfilling or rewarding. With a husband who traveled frequently and an extended family too far away to help, I felt claustrophobic and alone. I was a misfit in our small town, with my black outfits and clunky Doc Maarten boots (left over from grad school), drawing the curious glances of passersby. Women in the suburbs were blindingly colorful in their Lily Pulitzer dresses and rainbow shades of Patagonia fleece. I did my best to meet some like-

2

minded souls, but I grew tired of the local moms' group and conversations that centered around house remodels and summer camp plans. At night, I listened enviously as my husband relayed stories about the lunch he had with a CEO or the deal his firm was working on. I thirsted for adult conversation and a reason to use my brain again.

With each successive child, my desire to do something other than "mother" grew larger. Lord knows, I had enough to keep me busy with my charges, each of whom wanted all of me, all of the time. Who would shuttle them back and forth between basketball, Little League, ballet and swim classes if I were not there? Who would help them with their homework, give them a hug when they were sad, listen as they vied to recount the "best" and "worst" parts of their day?

But something inside me was unsettled. Maybe it was the expectation of professional success that comes with an Ivy League degree, or maybe it was just my own Type-A personality, but I felt that there must be more to life than what I was doing as a mother. If I had to pick up another Cheerio off the floor, I would blow my brains out!

After ten years of changing diapers and chasing toddlers, helping with homework and volunteering in the classroom, I decided to reach out to other women like myself to see how they were dealing with the disconnect between motherhood and professional ambition. I connected with former classmates, work colleagues, and friends both old and new. We talked on the phone, we emailed, we texted. Most of the women greeted my questions with great relief and a kind of confessional zeal as they recounted their struggles to reconcile the dueling demands of kids and career. Whether at work or at home, they reported feeling overwhelmed and exhausted, most, if not all, of the time.

I saw an opportunity.

By admitting they couldn't do it all, women could achieve a sense of freedom. By writing about it, they could achieve a sense of community. I put out a Call for Submissions for "true stories from the trenches of modern motherhood." Essays poured in from doctors, lawyers, bankers, teachers, writers, scientists, artists, stay-at-home moms, and women from all walks of life. While they had taken different paths, these women had one thing in common: despite their accomplishments and the many choices available to them, they recognized that doing it all – and especially doing it all *well* – was impossible.

*Torn* captures the voices of these women – a generation caught in the crossfire of kids, career, and family life. In a series of heartfelt and often laugh-out-loud essays, the book exposes the dirty truths of motherhood and the inevitable crises that life brings: battles with cancer, lost jobs and broken marriages, unplanned pregnancies and the heartbreak of infertility, and lots of "bad mommy" moments. In Katherine Shaver's "A Letter To My Daughter," the author launches into an examination of working mom guilt after she finds a Post-it Note stuck to her rear that reads, "Der Momy, I dont lik you anemore." In "Fluidity," Lydia Denworth discusses how raising a son with special needs derailed her career as a journalist but opened the door to a different type of writing, one which launched her career as a bestselling author. Tracy Thompson opens up about her struggle with debilitating anxiety and depression in "Balm" and shows how the moments of grace found in motherhood have helped keep her alive. In "Quartet," Courtney Williamson reflects on her undergraduate years at Dartmouth, where she raised a child in her dorm room while her peers went to fraternity parties. Jessica Scott, in "The Mommy Box," discusses the pain of missing her daughter's fifth birthday as she serves a tour of duty in Iraq.

As these stories illustrate, there is no perfect mother, nor is there a perfect balance when it comes to kids and career. Caught between the heady "have it all" idealism of our feminist foremothers and the rigid realities of the corporate world, women today are creating new paradigms to navigate the conflicting worlds of paid work and parenthood. While it is no longer unusual to see a successful executive, physician, professor or military officer who is also a mother, women are succeeding professionally not *because* of organizational and societal support, but *in spite of* it. They continue to break barriers by shattering stereotypes, discovering creative solutions for combining roles, and providing models for the next generation of women. In the end, these women – many of whom were brave enough to share their personal stories for this book – are playing an integral role in shaping what the future of motherhood will look like. Their voices take part in an emerging mothers' movement that is calling for better options for integrating work and family; greater respect for the social and economic value of mothers' work, paid or unpaid; and public policies that respond to the needs of working mothers and dual-earner couples. Their stories give us hope that, not too long from now, the notion of women feeling "torn" between family and career will be a memory of the past.

– Samantha Parent Walravens, Editor

# STELLA ON MOTHERHOOD

maybe goldfish
would have been a better idea
with her husband away so much
she could have handled goldfish on her own
goldfish never talk back
don't require self help books
on how to raise them right
birthday parties aren't a big deal
no homework     music lessons
parent-teacher conferences
and no driving around in endless circles
dropping off     picking up
getting them all to cooperate
into the van
out of the van
who's sitting where
no        goldfish are more settled
in their routine
don't demand   much
and if ever    fed up
flush them down the toilet
if a change of heart
quick trip to Walmart for replacement
it's just     that she'd miss
the sloppy kisses
mushy home-made birthday cards and
love ya   mom

– Joan-Dianne Smith

# PART ONE

# BALANCE, SCHMALANCE

ೞೞೞ

*No one could have taught me the most important lesson:*
*when you combine work and motherhood, there is no*
*balance.*

– Leslie Morgan Steiner

# FLUIDITY

*Lydia Denworth*

Fluid. This is how I sum up my life as a working mother. I'm not talking about the actual fluids that fill our lives as moms – apple juice, breast milk, tears, urine, projectile vomit – though it's surprising, now that I think about it, how well those liquids can sum it all up. Like the time I reached up from the couch to take a just-fed baby from my husband's arms and said baby spewed everything he'd just drunk into my face and mouth. Lessons: expect the unexpected, kids can go from adorable to disgusting in an instant, and it takes a long time to wash away the taste and smell of baby barf.

But that's not the kind of fluid I mean. I mean ever-changing like a river that begins as a stream high in a mountain and makes its way, eventually, to a wide flat delta where it joins the ocean. And it's not just the scenery that's changed along the way. As I've traveled along this river of parenthood, captain of a sometimes jolly, sometimes mutinous crew, I have made them switch boats practically at every bend.

Before I had kids, I thought the decision about work was a straightforward one – whether to work for pay (full or part-time) or stay home. Don't misunderstand. I did not think it would be easy to decide, or completely satisfying, whichever way I went, but I thought that was the basic choice. I would weigh all the usual considerations: income versus cost of childcare, desire to spend my days with my children versus desire to continue my professional life, and so on. I would make a choice and be done with it.

As I prepared to have my first child, I chose to take a long

11

maternity leave and then return to work. I assumed I'd do the same after the births of any other children I would be fortunate enough to have.

That's not how it worked out. In the eleven subsequent years, I have revisited that choice six times. I stayed home for a year. I worked part-time. I stayed home again. I worked full-time and then part-time and then full-time again. I have worked from home and from an office outside our house. I've also done a considerable amount of volunteer work.

I have had no help, a little help, and a lot of help with childcare. I have scheduled my life around pick-up and drop-off, and I have refused to schedule my life around pick-up and drop-off. I have used day care, babysitters, au pairs, housekeepers and after-school programs. I have my share of war stories from the clashing home and work fronts – like the day of a critical, impossible-to-reschedule interview when one son had pneumonia and the babysitter had the stomach flu. (Fortunately, and unusually, my husband was able to come home early that day.)

For the record, I am a journalist, able to work on a freelance basis. I have three boys, all school-aged, though the youngest is only in kindergarten as I write. One is hard of hearing and uses a cochlear implant and hearing aid. My husband works twelve-hour days; he is usually gone by six a.m. and home after seven p.m. He travels for work and often entertains clients in the evening. His comfortable income and inflexible schedule have affected my working life in two ways: I don't have to earn much, but I do have to be available whenever necessary. As a result, I have avoided having a boss or colleagues in an office expecting me to show up daily.

All the stopping and starting and adjusting of hours and help can sometimes put me in limbo – somewhere betwixt and between the stay-at-home and working mothers. Occasionally, I crave clarity, assuming it will sweep away all perceived problems and leave me feeling proactive, rather than reactive, and more in control. But I also recognize, when I'm feeling self-aware and forgiving, that each recalibration of our familial balancing act made sense. I changed my mind in accordance with whichever of the conflicting emotions and obligations familiar to every working mother dominated at the time.

When I quit work the second time, for instance, I had spent most of the previous year overwhelmed by the demands of a toddler, an infant and too much outside work with too little help. I was sure that I was doing neither my parenting nor my writing well. I thought the solution was more help, but then my third pregnancy came along unexpectedly quickly, so I went the other way – less work. A year and a half later, when our son's hearing loss was diagnosed, the hearing tests and doctors visits went on for months and took up several days a week. Although I had eagerly been looking forward to getting back to work right around that time, the fact that I didn't have to was fortunate.

Like many children, mine don't handle change all that well, so it's not surprising that the transition from one work routine to another has always been difficult. After more than three years staying home, my first step back into the working world was a journalism fellowship that consisted of two four-day sessions a few states away. It's a sign of how hungry I was for intellectual nourishment that the idea of sitting in conference rooms listening to PowerPoint presentations for a few days was as tantalizing as the smell of baking bread.

But then you might say I got burned taking the bread out of the oven. As the taxi waited to take me to the train station and I was double-checking my lists of instructions for the relatively new au pair, my youngest son, then two and a half, became hysterical. He ran to get his own shoes so he could come with me, then he struggled to get them on before the taxi could leave. Finally, with tears streaming down his red face, he stood forlornly on our stoop holding the shoes out toward me as I got into the taxi and wailing, "Mama. Mama. Mama."

Experts on separation anxiety say I did the only thing I could in that situation: I left. Drawing out the goodbyes only makes it harder for everyone. But telling that taxi driver to pull away was almost physically painful, and I was crying, too. Hours later, when I got to my conference, I was still shaken.

Even so, I knew in my gut that it was my turn to do something for me. I had devoted the last three and a half years of my life to my children. I adored them, but I was eager to return to work. Resentment and frustration had been building up in me over the last year, leaking out in my raised voice or lack of energy for playing. Four days away from them was not going to sever the bond between us. They would survive just fine – and did. And I would, too. (That new au pair, on the other hand, didn't last three months. Ah well. She wasn't cut out for three boys – or what I jokingly call Xtreme Parenting.)

The truth is, I've missed very little of my boys' lives. I know their friends and their teachers. I am able to attend just about every school function or performance (even if I've had to change plane flights to do it). Except for a one-year period when I often didn't get home until after they'd eaten, we've had most of our meals together and I've put them to bed more often than not. They talk to me about their hopes and fears, about fun and frustration, about best friends and "worst friends."

In those moments of craving clarity, I wrestle with the question of why I work at all if we don't absolutely have to have the money. Let's face it, if something has to go, giving the children back isn't an option. My answer is that I work because I like to work. At the risk of overstating the case, I even feel called to work. I write about subjects I believe are important, and about which I feel I have something to say. My volunteer work has centered on issues like education and community that I think are essential. I like to be engaged in the world in a more intellectual, professional fashion than day-to-day childcare allows. I like the challenge and sense of accomplishment that work provides. I found that when I went for stretches without working, I really missed it. And, to be honest, I was bored silly by playing the same game for hours with the kids when they were young. (As a friend put it, I'm not a great floor mom.) I believe the satisfaction I get from working makes me a better mother – less organized for sure, but happier.

As the mother of boys, I also feel a heavy responsibility to raise them to be good men who respect women. I want to be an example to them of all that women can do. Almost nothing satisfies me more than succeeding in that. When my oldest son was in second grade, he chose to interview me for his article in the class newspaper. At that point, I was president of our neighborhood civic association. His article began: "My mom goes to a lot of meetings." Oh boy, I thought. Here we go. But I was in for a pleasant surprise. The message of the article was that I was doing good work by contributing to my community. Even better was the day my first book arrived in the mail. The boys danced with joy in the kitchen, each hugging his own copy to his chest like it was treasure and saying, wide-eyed: "Wow, did you write every word?"

Very little has gone as I imagined it would back when I embarked on my first maternity leave. Working for yourself, for instance, does not always mean you are in control. I planned a maternity leave after the birth of my second child, but magazine articles I'd written months earlier went into the editing and production process literally the day I got home from the hospital.

Working from home has its advantages, but it has real disadvantages too. I always assumed it would be hard for the children if they knew I was in the house, but I found it was as hard for the babysitter as it was for me. If I could hear them arguing or crying, I felt duty-bound to investigate the problem. I've never forgotten the image one writer described of exiting her house in a suit and heels as if going to work, then sneaking around back to her office over the garage. Unfortunately, we live in the city and don't have a garage.

When I began writing that first book, I knew it would require copious research and considerable travel (back when I came up with the idea, I rather blithely assumed I would figure out how to do that). Furthermore, I had never written anything longer than a few thousand words. I couldn't imagine how I could fulfill my contract without renting an office and hiring a lot of help, which I did. That strategy worked in that I did the research and got the book written. The arrangement worked well. I left for work in the morning with the kids and returned in the evening. When I was at work, I was at work. When I was home, I was home. But I found I was uncomfortable with both the expense of this way of working and with the level of outsourcing required.

In addition, I've found that children need you more when they're older. Those were the wise words of a friend who is about five years ahead of me as a parent and she was absolutely right. Yes, they are gone for longer stretches of the day and don't need the same minute-by-minute caretaking, but the things with which they do need help feel bigger and more critical. A loving and capable caretaker can watch over a toddler on the playground, but who do you want to have on hand when a ten-year-old is upset about something he heard in the schoolyard about sex, or is mystified by math?

So here I am, at a bend in the river when I would have predicted I'd be full-steam ahead in work mode – kids in school, one book published, another on the way, new teaching responsibilities – and I'm switching to a slower boat. Although I know it will be harder to get work done, and that the economy is such that my income is increasingly more important, I gave up the office and much of my help. Am I working full-time or part-time? I couldn't say. I work when and where I can. I meet my deadlines either by being efficient or by staying up late. I'm with my kids when and where I can be. How delightful that they find Costco delightful!

I'm recalculating how to make it all work for the next school year. Some days the boys will go to after-school, some days I'll pick them up, and some days they will be shuttled to and fro by some new, as yet undiscovered and therefore still idealized babysitter. Making it work requires discipline, and that's something I wish I had in greater supply. But I have to believe I'll figure it out, mostly because I have in the past.

Between the last paragraph and this one, my cell phone rang. It was my oldest son, the very one who'd thrown up on me ten years earlier, now finished with his trumpet lesson. "Can you pick me up?" He was one block away – a block he travels by himself every day. "Do you need me to?" I asked, looking longingly at my computer. I was able, for the first time in days, to envision the end of this essay, and suspected that what he really wanted was for me to buy him a cookie at the coffee shop across the street. "No, but we've been having such nice conversations lately," he said. I closed the computer and walked up the block to meet him. He wouldn't have asked me if I hadn't been working at home; but then again, I wouldn't have been able to go.

Moments like that allow me to look back upstream and realize that perhaps I haven't been such an indecisive riverboat captain after all. You take on shipmates when you need them. You set sail when the wind blows. You can drift on a raft when the water is slow and shallow. In the rapids, you paddle like hell. The lessons are the same. Expect the unexpected. Embrace fluidity. Perhaps what matters most is that you've got a boat at all — and time to enjoy a conversation in it as you travel.

# DORA THE EXPLORER, MY BABYSITTER

*Carrie Lukas*

I must be the worst mother in the world.

I look at my two girls: Molly, three and a half, hair uncombed, lying half upside down on the couch; and Meredith, less than two, dressed only in a diaper and ratty coat that's more security blanket than proper apparel. They are half heartedly watching the television as I stare at my computer, focused on finishing my editing job before this episode of *Dora the Explorer* expires.

If anyone asks, I don't hesitate to tell them how lucky I am. And I mean it. I have what could properly be characterized as the best of both worlds. I'm a work-from-home mom who has been employed for many years by a worthwhile organization that appreciates my contribution. I've been able to continue working in a career I love, earning money, without giving up almost any hands-on time with my kids.

Sound perfect? I thought so. Even years before I became pregnant, I thought hard about what my ideal work arrangement would be after having a family. This was it.

I began working for the Independent Women's Forum, a Washington D.C.-based nonprofit group, in 2003. I was hired as a regular office worker. I showed up at nine, had a lunch break with my colleagues, and headed home around 5:30. There were meetings and receptions, but the bulk of my job was done in front of a computer.

That's what gave me my opening. After Molly was born in the fall of 2005, I made the case to my boss that I should be allowed to work from home full-time. The writing and editing I performed could be done remotely, and I would line up ad hoc babysitting to handle the sporadic meetings, media interviews, and events that required my actual physical presence. I argued that my two-year track record with the organization proved I was no slacker. I could be trusted with this kind of flexibility and had all sorts of ideas about how to measure my work so I could be held accountable. My boss and the board of directors most of whom were mothers themselves were quick to accept. They wanted to be as supportive as possible of a woman trying to achieve that much ballyhooed "work-family balance."

The news that they had accepted my proposal was an enormous relief. I didn't have to make the terrible choice between a career I loved and a baby I couldn't bear to hand over to another caretaker for so many of her waking hours. I could be both a full-time worker and a full-time mother.

And at first I really could. Newborns can be terrifying to care for. They are so fragile and mysterious, with their little cries and constant diapering needs. But they also sleep a lot. The three-hour intervals that switch almost regularly between sleep and consciousness make for some brutal nights, but leave ample time to get work done during the day.

My first few months back on the job went smoothly. I worked at night and during naps; I participated in conference calls and interviews over the phone. In the spring after Molly was born, I published a book, and the publicity department lined up dozens of radio interviews. That may sound glamorous, but most radio interviews are really just phone conversations broadcast to the world.

My job was perfect for me. I could stay in my typical get-up of jeans and a baby food stained shirt and still sound entirely professional over the phone. If Molly wasn't sleeping, I could stick her in front of the television and turn on *Dora*, or pop in one of the DVDs created to "educate" young babies. Did I feel bad about using the television as a babysitter? Of course. But given my situation, I felt it was a relatively harmless option.

Unfortunately for me, Molly was a precocious walker. She took her first steps early in her ninth month and was fully mobile a few weeks later. I hadn't properly thought through the full implication of that development when I plopped her in front of *Dora* in preparation for one of my fifteen-minute radio interviews. As always, I walked out of the family room into the kitchen – enough out of earshot that the interviewer wouldn't be able to hear the cartoon in the background. Yet a minute into the interview I began to hear alarming noises from the other side of the house. She was up! And far worse, I had somehow failed to properly hide the remote control (a magnet for just about any baby I've encountered). She had turned off her show and was starting to look for Mommy.

Mommy was struggling to sound upbeat and respond to the questions posed by the bubbly radio host while frantically thinking about where to hide. I ran to the bathroom and shut the door in time to keep Molly from physically reaching me. She sobbed on the other side of the door for the remainder of the interview, as I cowered in the bathtub trying to shield the phone from the noise.

Needless to say, it was far from my finest interview performance. I apologized afterwards to the booker who had set up the interview for the background noise that had marred my time on air. Professionally, it wasn't a big deal. Yet it brought home a reality that had been slowly creeping in: the hope that I could be both a full-time mom and a full-time worker without sacrificing something was a farce.

I can't do this, I thought to myself. I was awash in shame, both for letting down my employer and for allowing my young daughter to worry and cry on the other side of a closed door, while I completed a work task that in the larger scope of life was meaningless to me. Something had to give.

I began to seek more help in caring for Molly. I used my mother more often as a babysitter and began paying a neighborhood nanny to take her in for several hours so I could get work done without distraction.

That worked better until I got pregnant again. Baby number two added a host of additional complications. Less than a year after

Meredith was born, my husband accepted a position that would move the whole family overseas for a two-year stint. I welcomed the move as a chance to renegotiate my working relationship once again: no more meetings, fewer interviews, an even more flexible work life, and a significantly reduced salary. It was a compromise I could live with.

Now my third child sleeps in a bassinet as I type. I don't know exactly how his presence will change the delicate dance of mothering and working. Molly is in preschool in the morning, and Meredith, now two, will be joining her a couple days a week. I hope this will give me the time I need (along with help from Dad and a babysitter other than *Dora*) to get work done. I'll worry about when he starts walking when that time comes.

My four years of motherhood have taught me that there is no such thing as a perfect balance, particularly for those of us who have been both blessed and burdened with a first-rate education and a work life we care about, or need. We cannot help but think about the road not traveled. Stay-at-home moms will wonder about where their career might have gone if they had continued to work, and will encounter the economic vulnerability that comes with not working. Women who work full-time will feel the guilt of being absent for so many of the tender moments that childhood brings, as well as the pressure to try to "do it all." Those of us somewhere in the middle – part stay-at-home mom, part career mom – experience some combination of the two: regret about not doing more at work, regret about not being fully engaged at home.

It's no wonder that so many women seem to be looking for another solution. Women's magazines and television shows dissect the movement for "work-life" balance, and crusaders try to advance legislation to somehow make things easier on moms. Unfortunately, there is no set of policies that will solve the real root of the problem: we only have twenty-four hours in a day and can't be in two places at once. We have to make a choice about how to spend our time – indeed, how to spend our lives – and no one can make that choice any easier.

I'm happy with my choice. I'm also overwhelmed, anxious, exhausted, and worried that I'm not doing a good enough job making the most of my little charges' childhoods, let alone a good enough job at work. But I'm doing the best I can, cruising along at a steady pace on the road I've opted to travel.

# THE GOOD ENOUGH MOTHER

*Joana Jebsen*

Balancing career and motherhood reminds me of the proverbial angels dancing on the head of a pin – any imbalance and you will tumble off.

I started this balancing act early in my pregnancy. Because of an "incompetent cervix," I went into premature labor at twenty-one weeks. The doctors were able to stop the contractions, but they put me on strictly enforced bed rest for the remainder of my pregnancy. I had recently started a job at a pressure-cooker Internet startup, and I spent the next five months of my life negotiating contracts from bed, with a laptop on one side and cell phone on the other, trying to meet aggressive licensing targets. My husband would make me meals and put them in a cooler next to me. I was only allowed to get up to use the bathroom, a journey totaling five feet.

Every evening I put away my laptop and anxiously read pregnancy books, charting the number of weeks until I could safely give birth to babies whose lungs were developed enough to breathe. The twins arrived fifteen weeks later. After pushing out Baby A, I was told by my doctor to keep pushing. "Can't I take a break?" I begged weakly. "No," she said sternly. And that's when I first learned the truth about motherhood: there are no breaks.

My girls were beautiful and healthy. Baby A, with her wisps of dark straight hair, was destined to cuddle and dream; Baby B, strawberry blonde and equally adorable, came roaring out five minutes later – furious that she wasn't first and determined to make up for it.

Flash forward six months. I'm in a small hotel room in Mayfair, about to attend the London Bookfair. Exhausted and bleary-eyed from my transatlantic flight, I am desperate to pump the milk from my engorged, leaking breasts. They are enormous, like ripe cantaloupes.

"Would that be a humidifier, Ma'am?" asked the hotel manager, a man in his fifties with thinning black hair, large black glasses, and an impeccable British accent. He pointed at the large black box I was trying to plug in to the hotel wall socket. "No," I said. "It's a breast pump." I may as well have said it contained Anthrax. He retreated quickly toward the door. "I'll be right back, Ma'am," he said before fleeing.

The black box under question had defined much of my life since giving birth to my girls. Nicknamed "my breast friend," it looked like an object left behind by aliens – with suction cups, long plastic tubes and spare membranes. Despite numerous animated conversations with the breast pump representative stateside, the transformer they had sent me did not work in this London hotel. Luckily, Mr. Hotel Manager was able to overcome his antipathy. He returned with an even larger metal box, apparently a transformer of Herculean strength that could handle a breast pump, even if he couldn't.

I pumped before leaving for the conference, dashed back cross-town over lunch for another session with "my breast friend," had dinner with clients, and returned to the black box. I had become pretty savvy about pumping since returning to work. On my first day back after maternity leave, I remember searching our offices for a suitable "lactation chamber." True to dot-com style, our company had an open floor plan and few closed spaces. "Let's try the utility closet," the office manager had said. She opened the door to a windowless triangular-shaped room, trailing wires and cables. We ended up designating the first of two bathrooms as my lactation chamber. If I could lactate in a bathroom stall, I could lactate in London.

Four days later, I was back at the London airport for my trip home. In March 2001, there wasn't the intense post-9/11 scrutiny or laws limiting fluids – even human milk – to three ounces. But England was suffering from an outbreak of Hoof and Mouth disease, and travelers were forbidden from bringing dairy products in or out of the country. Somehow I had to persuade the airport official to allow me to bring my cooler filled with small freezer bags of milk back to the States. Fortunately the combination of "breast" and "milk" had the desired effect on the hapless British male official. He didn't want to know more. He wasn't fool enough to tackle a woman ready to fight to death for her offsprings' food.

My twin girls, now ten, often accuse me of loving my job more than them. As head of business development for a publishing services provider, I travel a fair amount, and it breaks my heart a bit each time I go. But when I'm not on the road, I work from home and do my best to be an active participant in my children's lives. I think of the frantic working mother in the British bestseller, *I Don't Know How She Does It*, who at midnight was distressing shop-bought fig tarts for a school fundraiser so they would look homemade. My version of this mad dance of working motherhood is baking brownies for a Girl Scouts event between conference calls ... trying not to forget they're in the oven ... hoping the calls don't go beyond the designated hour ... madly trying to carve the warm fudge into equal pieces ... struggling to get the confectioner's sugar to spread evenly on the still hot surface ... dreading the designer cupcakes the stay-at-home moms will bring. Only to find out that they are also too busy to bake from scratch and are bringing – oh, horror of horrors – store-bought cookies.

I've cobbled together a life as a working mom, and while it doesn't look so fancy, it tastes good enough.

# MOMMY CEO

*Sabrina Parsons*

My friends have nicknamed me "Mommy CEO" and joke about how I "do it all." If only they could see me racing into a morning meeting I scheduled, tired and lacking a shower because I was up all night with one of the kids, with spit-up all over my shoulder. If only they could see me driving like a mad woman to get to my son's preschool, having already shown up late to his doctor's appointment, while trying to finish a business call on my cell phone. I don't think this is the picture of Mommy CEO my friends have. Yes, if only I could do it all. That, however, would take a day with more than twenty-four hours.

I recently read an article that contained a survey asking working mothers to name their biggest work/family dilemma. According to this survey, there are four top challenges faced by working moms: needing to be two places at once, getting to work on time, never having enough time, and getting it all done. In my view, these are issues faced by all parents, not just moms. But there are things I have to deal with in the workplace that no man will ever face. No man will ever be in his office using a breast pump during a partner call, trying to get one more pumping session in, hoping and praying that the person on the other end doesn't recognize the telltale whirring sound in the background. No man will ever face the fear that their water will break all over the conference room floor during a critical meeting with potential investors. And very few men will ever face the reality that no matter how much government protection there is for maternity and family leave, there are some jobs that don't allow a three-month leave of absence.

I am the CEO of a software company where forty people depend on my leadership. Full maternity leave was never possible for me. I was fortunate in that I could bring my babies to the office for the first three months of their lives. But once they got mobile – and vocal – the jig was up. The toddler years are perhaps the most difficult to multitask work and mothering. I've had conference calls at home where I've had to run outside the house to find a quiet place to talk, watching my toddler nervously through the glass doors, hoping that he would continue to entertain himself and not get in trouble while I finished talking. On one important call, I actually watched my two-year-old through the glass doors as he painted one of our white dining room chairs with his non-toxic, "washable" paint. In a perfect world, we wouldn't need to care if a reporter from the *Wall Street Journal* hears kids in the background. But this isn't a perfect world. When my husband asked why I let my son paint the chair red, I answered that I was just multitasking.

Last night, as I sat in my boys' room at bedtime, I thought about how much I have on my plate, how much I am juggling, and the items that fall by the wayside: my blog, my workouts, my sleep. My wingspan is simply not wide enough. If you saw me sitting in their room, you could actually envision this "wingspan" – my arms stretched out wide between my sons' beds so they can each hold a hand as they fall asleep. It's a bad habit that I started, but they are still little, and I am a working mommy with enough mommy guilt to just let it go. So there I sit every night in the dark room, my arms just barely long enough to reach each of their beds and hold their little hands. Some nights my arms fall asleep, and my circulation gets cut off. Last night I sat there, hoping they would fall asleep quickly, and thinking that if my wingspan were just a little bit wider, I would be better off.

As that thought popped into my head (while I tried to scratch my nose with my knee), I realized that it was an apt metaphor for my life today. If only my wingspan were just a little wider, how much more could I accomplish every day? If only I could work a little bit faster, or the days were a little bit longer. What would that do for me? Right now I make critical time management decisions all day long until I go to sleep. In the morning: should I dry my hair or just run out with wet hair? At night, sitting quietly in the dark, arms outstretched: should I close my eyes, or think through our next email campaign or sales tactic?

Now the boys are asleep, and I consider whether to work out, catch up on email, or perhaps just sit and relax for a while. I realize that my wingspan will never be wide enough. The wider it gets, the more things I will try to accomplish every day. That is just who I am and how I operate. I think all those working mothers out there would probably nod in agreement. We can always work more, do more with our kids, organize and clean more, work out more, sleep more. Maybe we moms just need to relax and give in.

# HIGH HEELS AND HIGHLIGHTS

*Kathryn Beaumont*

At times, sitting at my desk with legal pads and case notes scattered about me, I envision myself comfortably garbed in yoga pants with a Starbucks in hand, strolling my daughter down the tree-lined sidewalk to the neighborhood playground. The vision is so seductive that I'm tempted to call up human resources and give notice. Instead, I straighten my pinstripes and head down thirty-three floors, plunk down $4.25 for a Venti soy latte, and gear up for another ten-hour day.

Before I became a lawyer, I took my two Ivy League degrees and worked as the following: an editorial assistant for a magazine; a reporter for a small-town newspaper; a hostess at a Mexican restaurant; a barista at a coffee shop; a nanny; a clerk at a fancy wine shop; a high-school English teacher; a stringer for a celebrity gossip magazine; a writer for my college's alumni magazine; an editor for a technology magazine; and a yoga instructor. Clearly, I didn't have a well-thought-out career path, other than that these jobs somehow supported my ultimate goal of being a "writer."

Needless to say, I never had much money. My first job out of Columbia Journalism School, as editorial assistant at a small magazine, paid $19,000 a year, on which I attempted to live in Manhattan and have a social life. That proved impossible, so I moved on. The years passed, and the jobs and the cities changed almost annually, yet I never made much more than twice my initial salary. My friends were buying houses and cars, and I was deferring grad school loans and charging uncomfortable amounts to my credit card each month. My friends had approached their careers with a bit more discipline: consulting firms, medical school, investment banking, law school. I, on the other hand, was trying to romanticize my career choices. Where my friends had "sold out," I was traveling the world! Living my dream of being a writer! Supporting my life with my jobs, as opposed to vice versa!

The problem was, my idealism never quite cured me of some upper-middle-class tastes. I liked a latte in the morning, nice clothes and fresh highlights. I also liked going out to dinner with my more gainfully employed friends, attending yoga classes, and buying designer bags. I wanted to embrace life as a starving artist, but I couldn't quite pull off dark roots or eating rice and beans.

These material superficialities aside, the truth also was that, as my thirtieth birthday approached, I found myself single and in a rather dead-end job. My friends' boring careers now seemed prudent and even enviable. Unless one possesses extraordinary talent or dedication (or a trust fund), none of which I enjoyed, being a writer is both financially frustrating and isolating. I was becoming more uncomfortable in my month-to-month existence. When, and how, would I be able to afford a home or a car? More important, I intended be a mother some day. If I never married and had to adopt a child on my own, how would I provide for that child?

So I went to law school – an idea I had toyed with over the past decade but also actively shunned in favor of what I romanticized as the more "difficult" and "true" path of being a writer. (Because anyone who couldn't figure out what to do after college simply went to law school, right?) Yes, I'd accumulate more debt, but if I worked hard, I would land a job with a good firm and make good money. I could get my hair highlighted whenever I wanted. I could drink soy lattes with abandon. I could wear sharp suits. My motives weren't entirely materialistic. As I rounded thirty, I had a deep understanding that I needed to grow up and think realistically about my future.

Shortly after starting law school, I met the man who would become my husband. Our angelic and entirely unanticipated baby was born the summer between my second and third years – just days after I had accepted a job with the biggest law firm in town. Most of the female attorneys I knew had planned their careers and families a bit more carefully than I had. They went from college straight to law school, spent a few years at a big firm, and then downshifted to a less-demanding position when they started having kids. This wouldn't be the case for me.

With some sacrifices, we could probably manage on one income if I truly wanted to stay home with my baby. The daydream was still there – the stroller, the lattes, the playground. But then I would think it through again: the walk to the playground would not be accompanied by a Starbucks because I'd feel guilty spending $4.25 on a fancy coffee; my hair would be mousy brown because highlights would be too expensive; my yoga pants would no doubt be ratty (why spend money on cute clothes?).

After nearly a decade of feeling like I wasn't living up to my earning potential, I enjoy being able to afford these luxuries. But more important, contributing to the support of my family brings me as much peace and fulfillment as would a day at the playground. I miss reading my daughter stories during the day and being there when she wakes up from her afternoon nap. But life holds too many surprises: a mid-life crisis, a heart-attack, a layoff in a faltering economy. Were something to happen to my husband, I could support us – all of us.

Though it breaks my heart a little when I leave my daughter – waving goodbye to me in the arms of her nanny – by the time I get to work, high-heels on, Starbucks in hand, gazing out past my computer screen at the sweep of the harbor thirty-three floors below me, I'm feeling pretty good. As difficult as it is not to be a part of my daughter's daily routines, I'm pretty sure she knows she is loved. What she probably doesn't know is that she is also provided for. On those mornings when I waver and wonder whether I'm doing the right thing, I think back over my colorful résumé of romantically low-paying jobs. And I go downstairs for another latte.

# NEED. TO. SLOW. DOWN.

*Sara Esther Crispe*

It was one of those mornings. The alarm clock didn't go off and of all days, this was the one when the kids had a class trip planned. At 8:30 a.m., I popped up in bed, realizing that their chartered bus had left about twenty minutes earlier. Frantic, I called the trip organizer, hoping to find someone who would be driving, and fortunately was given the phone number of a woman who she thought could take them.

Within exactly seven minutes the kids were out of the house with breakfast in hand. In addition, my two younger ones decided to come along for the ride. I had twelve minutes to make a drive that should take fifteen, but figured I would just make it.

With my eyes focused on the clock, I failed to notice the police car behind me. It was only when I heard sirens and moved to the side to let him pass that I realized he was not passing, he was pulling me over.

Now, I have never been pulled over for speeding, and this could not have come at a worse time. Without really thinking, I greeted him at my window with, "What did I do wrong? I am so sorry but I am really late to get my kids somewhere ..." to which he replied, "So that is probably why you were speeding ..."

Needless to say, so much for getting there in twelve minutes. Now I had to sit on the side of the road while he ran my license and papers. When he finally returned, he asked me if I knew how fast I was driving. Assuming this was a trick question, I told him I didn't, and asked him what he had clocked me at. He told me he hadn't clocked me, but that it was probably to my benefit, since I was definitely going well above the posted 25 mph speed limit.

As he handed me the ticket, he told me that he was actually doing me a favor since he was just giving me a fine and not a ticket with points. I thought of mentioning that it would be a bigger favor if he just gave me a warning, but decided against it. I ended up thanking him and apologizing for speeding in a fairly residential area. After all, I had four kids in the car and it was simply irresponsible. Not that I had been going dangerously fast, but nonetheless, clearly fast enough to warrant getting pulled over. He bid me farewell, and I was on my way, with four minutes left to get to my destination and a ten minute drive ahead. And a lovely $107.00 ticket.

Fortunately, my kids did make their ride, and I managed to adhere to the speed limit the rest of the drive. On the drive home, I started to contemplate the meaning of my ticket. After all, this Jewish month of Tishrei is all about working on oneself, judgment and atonement. Not believing in coincidence, I realized that my ticket definitely had greater meaning than not going a few miles over the speed limit.

My first reaction was that I had been given a ticket, a warning, but with no lasting repercussions other than a costly reminder that I should be more careful in the future. Knowing that I have a tendency to perhaps overlook the speed limit when I am in a hurry, I realized that there are numerous things in my life I ignore or neglect when something immediate is more pressing. In my mind, the speed limit seemed ridiculously slow for the major street where it was posted, but I began to think that there might be an important reason for it that I was not aware of. Maybe there had been accidents on that street in the past or it is a place where children often walk. And even if the speed limit truly was too slow for that area (after all, the limit on my residential street is 35 mph), it is a law, and one I am obligated to follow, whether or not I agree with it.

The fact that I was given a ticket but not given any points was a way of being told that this really was a warning, a wake-up call, a way of being made aware that I had to pay more attention and follow the rules, even the ones that seemed to make less sense to me. I had to be more careful, and I had to recognize that I am not in control of everything. There are guidelines to be followed, and no matter how late I may be, I have the obligation to adhere to them.

Thinking I had understood the deeper meaning behind my ticket, I called my husband to tell him what had happened and the lesson I had learned. His first reaction was to remind me that he had warned me not to speed when I left the house, because he knew I was running late. Yet, immediately after finding out that the policeman had not actually clocked my time, he took a very different approach.

Being the protective and supportive man he is, he decided that there was no way I could have been guilty and that perhaps I should fight it in court. He started arguing that chances were I was not speeding, that the police here have nothing better to do than give tickets, that the officer probably needed to meet his quota, and I was actually the victim in this case, because no one drives 25 mph on that street, and as long as I wasn't at least 10 miles over the speed limit, I should not have been ticketed.

As soon as he gave me his reasoning, I immediately became defensive as well. "Yeah, there is no way I was going that fast," I reasoned to myself, "How dare he give me a ticket after I told him that I had never been pulled over before and that I have a perfect record?" I started wondering if I hadn't really been singled out as an easy target. And then I realized that I could fight this. I could go to court. I could plead not-guilty and probably win, especially since he hadn't clocked me. I could get out of this.

But even as I thought it, I felt it just wasn't right. Yes, he probably did ticket me when I wasn't really going so fast, but I knew that I was most likely going faster than the speed limit. Yes, I knew I could probably get out of it, but was it right to do so if I had in fact been speeding? And, ultimately, was the fact that everyone else was speeding, that everyone else was doing something wrong, somehow a justification for my having done something wrong as well?

I realized that as much as my husband wanted to exonerate me, I needed to take responsibility. I had done something wrong, albeit nothing horrible, but simultaneously, I hadn't been given a horrible punishment. I felt that if I paid my ticket and admitted guilt, it would be a lesson, and one I would learn from and not soon forget. If anything, I started to realize that had the policeman just let me off, I may not have thought so long and hard about this and probably would not have taken it so seriously.

When I got home, I emailed my good friend, Amy, who more recently began to increase her observance of Judaism. She is an emotionally honest and sincere woman and has a way of seeing and stating things in a very direct manner. In my email, I mentioned my ticket and how I couldn't believe that of all days, I got caught this morning when I had to get the girls to camp.

I received a one-line email message back. It was so incredibly simple, yet profound in a deep and penetrating way. And it was a perspective that I had never thought of before. She wrote: "God is telling you to slow down in your life…"

Just slow down. How wise she was. I am always running. I am always moving. There is simply so much to do and so little time to do it. And it is easy to rationalize, to explain, to excuse because I am busy doing good things, positive things, which is why I can never slow down. But as much as you have to do, you have to keep the speed limit. You can't just move at a pace that is dangerous, even if your end goal is truly honorable. If your speeding causes you to crash, hurting yourself or another along the way, you will never reach your destination, and certainly not in time.

I thought about her words and even more, how I had my kids in the car when I was speeding. I began to think about all I do in a day and yet how much I also miss in their lives when I refuse to just do less. It is hard trying to be a mother and a wife and a friend and worker along with everything else all of us women do. But as another friend put it, when you have small children and life is so overwhelming, the days are truly long, but the years are short.

Sometimes, it feels as if you are tending to so many important details at the very same moment. After all, if you can make that much needed phone call while driving your kids to school, you are using your time well. A woman I know keeps a yellow sticky paper on her dashboard. It reads: "If you are talking on the phone, you are not talking to your kids…" How true. How very true. Yes, you might be getting your phone call out of the way, but if you are talking on the phone, and driving, and your kids are in the car, nothing that you are doing is getting 100 percent of your attention. You are cheating the person on the phone, you are cheating your kids, and you are not paying attention to the road ahead of you.

The days are truly long but the years are short. I started to think about all the times I answered an email while my children told me about their day at school or was too busy working to read them a bedtime story. And while at the time what I was doing seemed so necessary, so important, I was ignoring the posted speed limit for that particular time and place.

As I wrote out my check for my ticket and signed the line admitting guilt, I knew that I was admitting much more than merely driving over the speed limit. My ticket was a reminder that I need to reevaluate how I view the priorities and responsibilities in my life. But most importantly, it was a reminder that sometimes I just need to slow down…

*Originally published online at TheJewishWoman.org, 2007.*

# OF COURSE I WORK

*Susan Morse*

My mother owned a truly awful winter coat when I was young. It was a blue Eddie Bauer nylon parka, overfilled with down that poofed into a voluminous and shapeless mess. The coat sported a permanent coating of light brown dust, the accumulation of salt, sand and residue from small sticky hands.

My mother worked part-time as a lawyer throughout my childhood, at a time when it was unusual for women to practice law. Most evenings my brothers and I would join her in the kitchen while she cooked dinner – her maroon leather briefcase thrown onto the kitchen counter, her shoes lodged next to an overstuffed file cabinet, and her hideous blue coat still on her back. Tired and distracted, she would do her best to listen to the three of us as we vied to report the events of the day.

As a child, I don't remember minding that my mother worked outside our home. I was proud of her, even though fairly early on I realized that her income was not vital to our family's wellbeing, and that we might have even been losing money (figuring in the cost of child care) on a cash flow basis because of her job.

The apple doesn't fall far from the tree.

I started my career in a partner-track position at a big tax law firm. I arranged to go part-time after the birth of my first daughter, but my plans were foiled when I received a phone call from the IT department with "good" news: the wait list for smart phones had cleared, and a shiny new Blackberry was waiting for me in my office. I froze. I knew what the phone meant: checking email while at music class, being available to clients late into the night and all weekend, never being truly off duty. My idea of part-time work was inconsistent with a Blackberry-tethered lifestyle.

My fears were not ungrounded. The law, by nature, is a client-driven business, and what I thought would be the golden ticket of part-time employment turned out to be a fantasy. So I found something else – a job as a part-time, non-tenure track law professor, where there was no 24/7 availability requirement. I could do what I loved best – research, write and teach. My first published work as a professor was written when my youngest daughter was an infant and nursing through the night. After her 4 a.m. feedings, I would force myself out of an oxytocin-produced haze to sit down at the kitchen computer and work until the rest of the family woke up. My husband kept things together in the irritable hours that followed and never failed to support me in my career choice, even though my job wasn't paying enough to cover the expenses incurred.

This year I transitioned into a full-time academic post that offers the opportunity for promotion and career advancement that my previous job lacked. Yes, it takes me away from my daughters more than I would like, but I have learned from my mother that I have a responsibility to myself and my daughters to work – to provide a living, breathing example of a woman's ability to pursue a career and motherhood and reap the benefits of both.

My mom recently celebrated her fortieth anniversary with the same government legal group she worked for when I was a kid. She sent out a family email reporting that she had been promoted to a position one notch below her boss's old job. She was proud, and I was proud of her. Working was not always easy on her or our family, but I understand now the sense of independence and fulfillment that her job gave her, a benefit that has lasted long after her children graduated and left the house. As she reminds me today, it's okay to miss a few basketball games or to skip the toddler ballet classes that don't fit into our family schedule. The kids will turn out fine. I'm living proof.

I brought one of my daughters to work with me when I was in a pinch not too long ago. She sat at the back of the classroom, her nose buried in a science fiction novel, as I enthusiastically taught a class on business tax law. She looked up every now and then with a look of utter boredom on her face. After class, I told her about the time my mom brought me to work with her. Nana was on a business call and I peed in my pants, right there in her office, because I didn't know where the bathroom was. It could be worse, I explained.

There are many evenings when I wish I were not racing to cook dinner with my work clothes pinching at my waist, hurriedly helping my children with their homework so I can climb into bed and spend a few minutes alone with my husband before we fall asleep. But when I think about quitting, it's like contemplating the amputation of my legs. For me, work is dignity. It is breathing. It is a safety net for the future if something should happen to my husband or my marriage. It's an example for my daughters, who will most likely experience the same juggling act in their own lives.

In an effort to cheer me up after a long day recently, my nine-year-old wrote on a piece of construction paper, in her best cursive handwriting:

> Mom:
> chauffeur
> chef
> law expert
> teacher
> reader
> computer whiz
> cleaner
> shopper
> swimmer
> gardener
> home remodeler
> and more!
> Always On Top Of It.

Maybe my kids do get it. I smiled and put the note in my pocket.

# PART TWO

# GOT GUILT?

ೞೞೞ

*Guilt: the gift that keeps on giving.*

– Erma Bombeck

# LETTER TO MY DAUGHTER

*Katherine Shaver*

Dear Laura,

Last night, as I was cleaning the kitchen – long after your bedtime – and trying to ignore your "I'm not going to bed!" protests, I felt a little hand press firmly against my right butt cheek. I turned around to find a yellow Post-it Note stuck to my rear just as I caught a glimpse of you running around the corner.

It read, "Der Momy, I dont lik you anemor."

You are two weeks shy of six years old. The dog-eared parenting books on my nightstand describe you as "temperamental" and – how's this for spin? – "spirited."

It has not been lost on me that you get more spirited on the three days a week when I go to work. I arrive home exhausted, my tires practically screeching into the driveway to meet the babysitter while answering deadline questions from my editor by cell phone. These are the nights when bedtime feels rushed. I snap more easily, and you stretch out your arms from bed and cry, "Mommy, I miss you!" Scratch another mark in the "I suck as a mother" column. The other night, I actually went online and ordered a children's book titled, *Why Can't You Stay Home With Me? A Book About Working Mothers*. I ignored another offering titled, *Why Mommy Stays Home – We Chose You*.

For the past six years, I thought I had it all worked out. Sure, my life has felt like a house of cards that comes crashing down whenever our babysitter cancels, or you or your three-year-old brother spikes a fever and wants Mommy as much as grape-flavored Tylenol. For the most part, however, life has chugged along pretty smoothly. I have had few serious regrets. I know that I am a kinder, more patient, and – dare I say it – happier mom because I have a life outside of motherhood.

Then, this. Your outstretched arms. Your tantrums. Surely they must have something to do with your adjustment to kindergarten. But I'm starting to get a big-time case of the guilties.

After you were born, I spent the last weeks of maternity leave worrying. I had spent my entire life doing what I was "supposed" to do, but suddenly I didn't know what that was anymore. I had thought that I would believe so strongly in the importance of raising a child that my decision to quit working would be clear cut. My own mother had punted on her career as a pediatrician – just a few years after slogging through medical school and her residency – to raise my three siblings and me, and I have never once doubted that she is one of the most intellectual and interesting women I'll ever know. She raised four reasonably happy and successful adults. Surely, I thought, my father's untouchable work ethic and my mother's sacrificial devotion lay behind that.

So why couldn't I do the same? Because one day at a play group, as we mothers cooed over our babies, I felt my mind begin to dissolve. The discussion had focused once again on formula versus breast milk and co-sleeping versus crying it out. I turned to the woman next to me with a question that always feels a bit verboten among stay-at-home mothers : "What did you do before you had kids?"

"Oh," she said, absent-mindedly. "I was a social worker for juvenile delinquents in the Bronx."

Suddenly, I wanted to chat.

I tried to chalk up my desire to continue working to higher ideals – that I owed it to feminism, that I should show my daughter how to make her own way, that I wanted the financial freedom to go shoe shopping without feeling like I would have to justify every purchase to my husband. I told myself I needed to use my Princeton degree and honor the thirteen years I'd spent working late nights and weekends to land a job at a prestigious newspaper. I never took it for granted what a luxury it was to have a choice. I knew that most working mothers needed to support their families. With our savings and some careful budgeting, your father and I could have made it work on one salary, at least until you and your brother reached school.

Toward the end of my maternity leave, I realized I had started looking for ways simply to get through the day until your dad walked through the door and I could read the newspaper and have a glass of wine. I worried that a world I had covered for almost two decades as a curious tell-me-all-about-it journalist would become too small, even claustrophobic. I had always assumed that, like my mother, I would want to be home with my children full-time. But when I stopped beating myself up long enough to accept the hard truth, I knew I couldn't do it very well for very long. I also felt certain that if I were happy, my children stood a better chance of being happy, too.

My own mother sealed my decision. When I told her about my struggle, I was surprised to hear her say that she'd always wished she had gone back to work part-time after having kids. She shared the sting of attending Cornell University Medical School reunions and seeing classmates who had become standouts in their fields. She said she'd always been a tad jealous of a female neurologist who had worked part-time while raising a family. When that woman's children were grown and gone, my mother said, she had something left for herself. Still, she had believed that continuing her medical career would have made it impossible to be the kind of mother she wanted to be. She didn't want to miss anything, she said. She wanted to ensure that her children got to Brownie meetings and ballet classes. Stay home with your kids because *you* want to, she told me, but only if being a full-time mother is a life experience that *you* want. Don't do it for your children. If you do, you might end up resenting them.

The day before I returned to the office, I spoke with a friend who also works part-time and is an involved and loving mom. She heard my voice quiver with last-minute uncertainty. "Oh, it's so much better than you'd think," she said in a conspiratorial half-whisper. "You can go to the bathroom whenever you want! You can drink coffee and check your email – at the same time!"

The truth is, I liked being back at work. (Do "good mothers" admit this to anyone but their closest working mom friends?). Sure, I could get choked up just glancing at your baby photos tacked above my desk. But I still feel a bit like Clark Kent transforming in the phone booth when I swap out the crayons and sippy cups in my purse for ballpoint pens and lipstick. I would deeply miss the time I spend talking to grownups about the world beyond The Wiggles. I'm proud that my part-time salary still covers our mortgage. Ironically, my job reviews are the best of my career. You can get a lot done when no one is chanting "Mommy Mommy Mommy Mommy" in your face. But I have also mommy-tracked myself. I watch less experienced reporters leap frog over me because they can – or will – devote seventy hours a week to covering the White House and can hop a plane at a moment's notice to reach the latest earthquake. I don't get paid for the days "off" when I find myself oh-so-glamorously perched on our powder room toilet to conduct brief phone interviews, hoping the overhead fan drowns out the screams of you and your brother fighting.

Still, I am grateful for bosses who give me the flexibility to work harder over fewer days. I relish my time at home because it is not constant. At a less frenetic pace, I morph into a mom who helps out in the school cafeteria and ferries her kids to gymnastics. I have never resented you or your brother, because I didn't give up the professional life that makes me tick. I have hamstrung my career, but I can live with the scales tipping your way.

When it comes time to make your own decision – and I do hope that you, too, will have the luxury of getting to choose – be honest with yourself. Ignore those who tell you why you "should" work or not. Like me and my own mother, you will be able to argue both sides. You must strike your own balance, even an imperfect one. It won't be easy. I still struggle with both the working mother's guilt of not being home to meet the school bus and the stay-at-home mother's fear that my professional worth might never recover from stepping off the traditional career path. Remember, it's when you think you've got it all figured out that your babysitter will quit without warning or you will find an angry Post-it Note stuck to your rear.

But it is worth it. Three weeks have passed since I began this letter. Last week, it was your sixth birthday. I had planned the entire day – one of my work days – around being in your classroom at 2:30 p.m. to help hand out your birthday cupcakes. It required slinking out of the office and driving like mad for thirty-five minutes. I had intended to leave the school immediately after the birthday celebration and rush back home to finish my work. After all, I had a story deadline hanging over my head and too little time on my side. Then you pleaded with me to stay. With typical six-year-old reasoning, you wanted to take the school bus home with your friends but also wanted me to put you on the bus at school and then drive home to meet it. I resigned myself to working late after you were in bed, and I stayed. As you sat on the colorful carpet with your classmates waiting for your bus to be called, you pulled a little pad of princess paper from your pink backpack and wrote intently. Walking hand-in-hand out to the bus, you gave me the note: "I love you momy," it said, "so, so mush."

With much love,

Mommy

# THE MOMMY BOX

*Jessica Scott*

My daughter turns five today. Instead of being there to watch her blow out the candles on her birthday cake, I'm in the hot, dusty city of Mosul, Iraq, serving a year-long tour of duty as an officer in the U.S. Army. Most days, the pain is buried behind meetings and maintenance and drills, but sometimes, the pain breaks out. Days like today, when all the mommy stuff breaks out of the box I've mashed it into, I have to stuff it. It's the only way to cope with the pain of the missed milestones, like first steps and first days of school. I have to lock them up tight. Tight enough that I don't have to admit how badly it hurts. Tight enough that I'll go through an entire day of meetings and briefings and answering emails without once thinking about my children. I try not to talk about my family with anyone other than my husband, because at the end of the day, I know that opening the mommy box will unleash a maelstrom of feelings and I have a job to do. I can't do that job if I'm blinded by tears. There have been a few cracks this year. The first time was back when the swine flu broke out. I was alone in my trailer, watching news anchors from around the world talking about this latest "apocalypse." The hyperbolic stories and over-inflated statistics about the suddenness of the strike and the lethality of this particular virus hit me hard.

I was already raw from reading *The Shack*, a book about a guy whose child is murdered (not a good choice for a mom who's separated from her kids by oceans and deserts). Rationally, I knew that being away from my kids had absolutely no impact on whether they got sick, and with my mom as a caretaker, I knew they couldn't be in better hands. But rational thought didn't stop the panic attack – the panic attack that I had quietly, by myself, and told no one about until well after the fact.

The next crack was on my daughter's first day of kindergarten. I bawled like a baby listening to her tell me about her first day and hearing the exhaustion in her little words. Because she was living with my mom, she was attending the same school I did when I was a little girl. I recalled my first day of school – the little green windbreaker I wore and the ˙sticker with my name on it. I remembered being scared to get on the bus, but my mom was there with me, holding my hand, taking my picture, and making it into a big, fun adventure. Now, twenty-plus years later, my mom was there again at the bus stop, making everything okay for my daughter, because I couldn't be there for her.

The hardest thing about being away is knowing that my daughter will remember. She'll remember me not being there to walk her to the bus and wave goodbye at the small, tinted window. She'll remember blowing out the candles of her birthday cake with her grandmother taking pictures, not me. Although I have been there for my youngest daughter's three birthdays, between my husband's and my deployments, we've missed more than half of her life. My mother was the one who took charge of the potty training and who was there to watch her first steps. She's the one who held my girls when they got sick and who brought my little one to the doctor when she sliced her thumb open.

We can talk about the sacrifices military men and women make for their country, but at the end of the day, it's personal. It's about missed birthdays and Mother's Day without Mommy and tears on the first day of school when every other mom but you is there to kiss their kids goodbye. It's about the pain of not being able to cradle your sick child, and the sadness of having to experience the most precious moments of your kids' lives through pictures and long distance phone calls.

Last night on Skype, my three-year-old crossed her arms, dropped her little head and whimpered,

"Mommy, I want you to come home."

There's nothing quite like hearing your kids hurting and knowing there's nothing you can do about it. What three-year-old is going to understand the Army assignments process and war and the myriad of other reasons you can't come home right now? All I wanted to do was hold her tight and feel her breath on my neck. I wanted to brush my five-year-old's hair from her face and listen to her tell me how she learned what a veteran was in school the other day. I wanted the aggravation of getting them to bed on time and the hugs and kisses first thing in the morning. I wanted it so goddamned bad, but there was nothing I could do to make the time go by faster so that I could be with them again.

I put on a brave face for the camera and distracted them with promises of Texas Roadhouse steaks and a phone call the next morning. I fought hard to keep the lid tightly closed on the mommy box. My girls didn't need to see my emotions bubbling beneath the lid. They needed to know it was going to be okay.

I hope today that my daughter has a happy birthday. I'm looking forward to seeing the pictures and hearing her tell us about it. Most of all, I'm looking forward to being home. To taking my kids to school and the playground, making them dinner, and reading them bedtime stories. To experiencing the joy that comes from the mundane tasks of motherhood.

Happy Birthday, Baby. Mommy will be home soon.

# COMING HOME

*Jessica Scott*

Three weeks ago, I walked into my mother's foyer, greeted by cries of "Mommy, Mommy!" and hugged my daughters close for the first time in over six months.

In that moment, I was Mom again. I know that sounds off. Just because I spent a year in Iraq didn't mean I wasn't a mom while I was gone. In my heart and soul, I still worried about my kids; I still missed them. But I didn't have the day-to-day things that make me Mom in my kids' world. And in that precious instance, I had no idea just how hard it would be to come home again.

Coming home this time around was not as simple as picking Daddy up on the First Cavalry Division's parade field. Coming home this time involved figuring out what it meant to be a parent again. In my kids' case, we had taken away their home and their pets, their daycare and all the reminders of their daily life with us. Our animals, too, had to move in with other relatives for the duration of the year.

I've always been an emotional parent. But this week, when I took my oldest daughter to her first day at her new school, she clung to me, sobbing that she didn't want me to leave her. It was only school, but in her world, it might as well have been another year. She cried. I cried. And I looked at her teacher, a woman who had just met me the day before, and admitted through my tears that I did not know what to do.

It's a hard confession to make. What kind of parent doesn't know what to do when their child is upset and crying? What kind of mom doesn't know what her kids' favorite food is, or what to do when they are acting out? I didn't know how to deal with my child's separation anxiety. Nor did I know how to respond when my kids got angry and said things like, "I don't love you" and "I want Grammy." The hardest to hear was when my daughter told me, "You don't love me anymore," at a rest stop in New Jersey.

I have uprooted my children's lives more than once and left them with an aching suspicion that Mommy and Daddy will leave again. The guilt I feel for putting this burden on them colors my decisions on how I interact with them. I know there will be consequences down the road.

When I left for Officer Candidate School, my youngest was just shy of seven months old. I was in Fort Benning, my kids were in Maine and my husband was in Iraq. It was my first taste of what life as a military mom was truly like, but I had no idea how hard it was going to be to deploy and come home again. I knew my mom was taking good care of my kids. Still, nothing could have prepared me for the heartbreak I felt when I watched my baby crawl after her grandmother, calling her Mommy.

So often in military families, when Dad comes home from deployment, Mom has been there holding things down. There's a transitional period, but life has only been missing a single piece, instead of being uprooted entirely. I'm not saying that dads who deploy don't have transitions to make when they come home. But when both Mommy and Daddy are gone, the impact is different. It's harder on me emotionally in some ways because I've been the stability in our children's lives for the last two deployments. I've always known what to do with them.

But there I was, just days before, standing in the hallway of my daughter's school, surrounded by seventy five-year-old kids, crying because I didn't know what to do.

Thousands of moms who are coming home from Iraq and Afghanistan will feel the pain of their infant children calling someone else Mommy because they were babies when their moms left. They will feel the helplessness of not knowing how to handle a tantrum and the awkwardness of not knowing what their children like to eat. And, if they choose to remain in the Army, they will anticipate the fear of the next deployment, knowing that as soon as they figure out what normal is, their families will be uprooted once more.

I know what it feels like now to become a mom again. And I know the fear of deploying again or taking my children from their home and uprooting their lives once more. It's the life I lead, the life I chose. The life of a mom who is also a soldier.

My choice, however, does not make today's pain any easier to bear.

# CUPCAKE CRAZY

*Liesl Jurock*

A t 1:30 in the morning, I threw down my Rainbow Chip frosting-covered spatula. This could not be the best way to frost cupcakes; it was so messy and uneven. I pried open my laptop with my free elbow and Googled "how to frost a cupcake" with my two clean fingers. After viewing two video tutorials, I realized I was doing it just fine. I returned to plopping icing on each mini-cupcake, muttering angrily under my breath about the fact I couldn't equally distribute the bits of rainbow sprinkles amongst the thirty cupcakes.

Somewhere in the back of my mind, I knew I'd gone a little cupcake crazy. But over the past few hours, nothing else had mattered. My little boy was turning two, and I was following the unspoken rule of bringing cupcakes to daycare on his birthday. I'd never made cupcakes before, so I figured that was causing me a certain illogical level of anxiety. The fact that I was making two different Martha Stewart recipes for my son's two-year old classmates should have clued me in to the idea that I was taking this a little too seriously.

I remembered the last daycare party where one of the parents walked in with a tray of brightly decorated, freshly baked cupcakes, while the rest of us brought in store-bought snacks. The mom beside me muttered, "Boy, some people have a lot of time on their hands. I work full-time!" I nodded in agreement. Something about the table of treats in front of us definitely signified some kind of measure of our motherhood. I wasn't sure if my plate of crackers and cheese scored me points on the "good mom" scoreboard or the "bad mom" one. (I did slice the cheese and plate the crackers, and they were healthy, but there was nothing homemade about them!) But by the end of the party, the verdict was clear. Our toddlers had devoured the tray of cupcakes, their shirts covered in blue frosting, while the rest of us brought home leftovers. Suddenly, developing the cupcake-making skill became as important to me as learning to nurse my baby had been. It seemed as essential to my mothering repertoire as lullabies and kissing "ow-ies." I decided that at the next daycare event, I wanted to be the mom whom parents made snarky comments about. And I wanted to retort, "Yeah, well, I work full-time too!"

So, it was with great pride that I walked into daycare with my tray of cupcakes (and my son). His caregiver was too busy to be impressed, but the kids jumped up to sneak a peek. I excitedly told them, "You'll eat cupcakes with Lucas later." After settling Lucas in with his slippers and a truck to play with, I did my customary squat down to his level and told him, "Mommy has to go now." That was always the crucial moment that could go either way. Some days, he barely glanced up from his toy, whispering "bye bye, Mommy." Other days, like today, the opposite happened. He clutched onto my shirt, leaned all his weight into me, crying, "No Mommy go! No Mommy go!" Worse, his appeal was coupled with, "Mommy eat cupcakes with Lucas later!"

My heart was in my throat as I said, calmly, "Mommy won't be there when you eat cupcakes. Mommy has to go to work. You get to play here with your friends." I plastered a smile on my face and backed away a little, as the daycare staff moved in to comfort him. I stood up, allowing him to fall into the arms of the woman who would take care of him instead of me. As I bolted toward the door, I heard her saying, "Want to help me get our snack ready? We're going to have your cupcakes and sing Happy Birthday Lucas!" His screams died down, his interest diverted toward helping her.

My emotions did not die down as easily. I climbed into my car, put my head down on the driving wheel, and allowed the tears locked in my throat to release. But the sound of his "no Mommy go" reverberated in my head. When I finally put my hands on the steering wheel to start driving, I saw they were shaking. What am I doing? How can I leave him? How can a bloody meeting be more important than him? How can this job take priority? I found myself, not for the first time, considering handing in my resignation.

But at least he had my cupcakes. They were something I could give him. And suddenly I understood why I had been so obsessed about making them perfect. They had to be good enough to supersede the guilt I felt over not being there. Despite my love for him, the fact remained I was choosing work over my child.

Being a "working mom" made me the envy of some of my thirty-something pre-children female colleagues. I embodied their dreams; they looked at me and thought I had it all. And sure, I felt proud of what I'd achieved that past year – becoming a mother, getting a promotion, and finishing my master's degree. But often I wanted to scream to them, "Do you have any idea how hard this is?"

I wasn't talking about the work itself, but about the sacrifices. Staying late for a meeting meant I wouldn't see my son before he went to bed. When I indulged in chitchat around the water cooler, it meant I'd need to wake up at 5:30 a.m. the next morning and log in to my remote desktop to get caught up. When I got sick, I didn't get to rest until Lucas did. When I chose to talk to my husband, I sacrificed sleep. When we both tried to get enough sleep, it meant we skipped any chances for sex. I negotiated these things all day every day and finally realized … you could not actually have it all. You could have bits here and there at different times, but everything was at the cost of something else.

Still, I got to do this. I got to choose this. My counterparts sixty years ago were not so lucky. Even my own mother's generation was more likely to choose to stay home. Now there was a romanticism attached to stay-at-home motherhood that was about as true as my "you can have it all" narrative. Either way, as mothers at either end of the spectrum, our choices trapped us in different ways. My stay-at-home friends felt imprisoned, as if living Groundhog Day over and over. As a "working mom," I felt trapped on a hamster wheel, running the rat race of life and catching only glimpses of it as it went by.

But ten minutes into work, sitting in a fast-paced meeting, I remembered why I was there. I remembered why I chose this. I loved interacting with colleagues who shared my values and with students who were eager to learn from me about projects that were fun and challenging. I loved creating programs that made a difference. And I loved getting paid for it all. Yet, what was I missing as a result of my choice?

I excused myself from the meeting just before 10 a.m. and snuck back into my office, closing the door behind me. I logged on to the webcam of the daycare and squinted to find Lucas on the blurry screen. I saw him trailing after his favorite caregiver, and I blessed her kindness to him. Soon all the kids were being seated and cupcakes were being passed out. I couldn't hear anything with this webcam, but I could see all their little mouths moving, so I imagined them all belting out "Happy Birf-day" to Lucas. I whispered along.

I opened my lunch bag and pulled out my Tupperware container where my gooey little cupcake sat. I admired its perfection; it could be in Martha's magazine. On the screen, Lucas and his friends inhaled their cupcakes, smearing frosting all over their little faces. I joined in, ripping my perfect cupcake from its paper and devouring it whole. It wasn't the same as being there with them, but it was something. And in a life where you try to have it all and know you can't, you learn to take what you can get.

# Moms Just Can't Win

*Shelby Hogan*

L et's talk about Mommy Guilt. You know, that little voice inside your head, or from other people, that tells you that no matter what you do, it's not quite good enough. We all live under the specter of Mommy Guilt. Because let's face it: sometimes we moms just can't win.

Take the working moms versus stay-at-home moms. Working moms? What terrible people! If they loved their children, they'd eat ramen noodles every day and stay home to nurture their children in the way only a mother can! The moms who actually choose to work so they don't lose their sanity – how self-indulgent! The stay-at-home moms? How beatific, the self-sacrifice required to surround their children with love and care 24/7. What do they mean when they say they are bored and would love some adult conversation that doesn't involve discussing sleeping or pooping issues? If they loved their children, why on earth would they say something like, "I'd kill for a little time for myself"? Don't they know that there are working mothers out there who would love to be in their position? What's wrong with them?!

Like I said: working or not, we just can't win. It's Mommy Guilt in action, rifling out its ammunition in a devastating spray of "shoulds" and "shouldn'ts." Working moms: you should stay home with your children. Stay-at-home moms: you should be grateful and not complain. Working moms: you should do all of your parenting yourself and not leave it to some daycare worker. Stay-at-homers: you should put your children in preschool or a group setting, lest you raise some kind of weird, maladjusted freak who can't make friends or get along with anyone else.

Mommy Guilt. It's pervasive. Just sit and think for a moment about your kids. Count how many times the words "should" or "shouldn't" pop up in your daily lingo. Right now, I'm on the couch typing away on my laptop while my little guy is in the Pack 'n' Play, gazing rather dumbly at the carrying bag that came with some expensive blocks (which he just threw out in favor of the bag). I notice the dull, rather unintelligent look in his eyes. Shouldn't I be reading to him or practicing rolling a ball back and forth, which the book says he should be able to do but cannot at this point in his development, probably because he spends too much time in the Pack 'n' Play fiddling with the carrying bag instead of the expensive blocks? I'm getting ready to feed him some lunch, which I should have started already, but haven't. When I throw stuff on his tray, it really should be fruits and veggies I grew myself, organically, in our back yard. I also should be engaging him with eye contact to work on his language development skills instead of taking the opportunity to fold some laundry or do the dishes (which really should be done already). Oh, and did I mention that my little guy doesn't eat with a spoon very well? Why? Because he makes such a mess of it that nearly nothing goes into his mouth and it all ends up either in his hair or his sleeves or on the floor or inside the dog. Of course, if I take the time I should to teach him this valuable skill, he'll be far less likely to go to college eating like a caveman.

Wow, seven "shoulds" in a single sitting, most of which I will not follow through on anyway. A+ Mommy!

Now honestly, I can't bring myself to feel terrible about every one of those things. He'll get it eventually. Much of the time, I'm pretty good at managing the Mommy Guilt, recognizing it for what it is: total crap. But there are other times when the Mommy Guilt stays with me. When it really does make me feel like I'm not quite good enough. Did you know that a woman can have postpartum depression for a full year after her child's birth? Nothing feeds depression like a big old dose of Mommy Guilt.

I look back at my little guy. He doesn't use two-word sentences like the pediatrician asked about, but the few words he has, he uses wisely. "Da Da!" he says every time he sees a dog. "Da Da! Woo Woo!" goes his barking imitation. And more recently he has added "Arf Arf!" and "Wow Wow!" to his repertoire. The kid can't say Mommy or Daddy, but he barks like no other baby I've seen. Take that, Dr. Know It All!

No, my little guy doesn't do a lot of things the books say he should, but he does plenty else. Like when I tried teaching him sign language but gave up after a few weeks because I felt like an idiot talking to myself. Two full months later, I went to take off his bib at breakfast and looked down to see him frantically signing "more, more" completely out of the blue. And it wasn't a fluke. He had stored it away in his brain and whipped it out when it was truly crucial. Not only that, but he'd completely specialized the sign to mean "more fruit." Often his sign for "more" is accompanied by an expression that clearly says, "Hey, people! What's a guy gotta do to get an orange around here?"

So I say, "To hell with you, Mommy Guilt! To hell with you, culture of 'perfect parenting'! To hell with you, 'Should' and 'Shouldn't'!"

I am a mother, and I am more than good enough.

# MOTHER'S DAY IS NOT FOR WIMPS

*Cathleen Blood*

I sit up and fluff my pillows, preparing for my traditional Mother's Day breakfast-in-bed. Dad and the kids have been busy banging kitchen cupboard doors for the past half hour, but now all is quiet. My husband arrives, carrying a tray laden with coffee, a ginger scone, and a random assortment of flowers and branches from the garden, courtesy of my daughters who trail after him. My son loiters awkwardly by the bedroom door. The girls climb onto the bed, snuggling up like cats.

And so begins my annual moment in the sun.

My daughters present me with their homemade cards. (My son hands me a Post-it-Note, saying he will, without fail, deliver a card by the end of the day. Knowing my son, I save the Post-it.) One card is shaped like a flower. A single word is carefully printed on each petal. They are nice words. There is, however, an abundance of spelling errors, which I wisely choose to ignore. (I am an especially thoughtful mother, I think to myself.)

"This is very clever," I say to my youngest. Then I read the poem aloud …

> My Mom
>
> My mom is always helpful.
> She is so Thoughtful.
> My mom gives us everything we need.

She is Motherly.
My mom is always there when I need her.
She is very Caring.
My mom owns a big business.
She is Hard Working.
My mom has many rules that you have to follow.
She is Strict.
My mom always likes to try new things.
She is Interesting.
I LOVE MY MOM!

I well up, and my daughter smiles up at me with her wide-set hazel eyes. She is pleased. Scoring a tear on Mother's Day is a home run.

"I had to make most of it up" she says matter-of-factly. "The teacher made us all make cards at school. It was hard to think of enough nice things to say, so I copied some from Monica. And I didn't write about all the bad stuff," she adds proudly.

My warm buzz fades. So much for my moment in the sun. Darned kids. How can I maintain the delusion that I am an amazing working mom in the face of such honesty? And because I'm competitive, I have to wonder, is Monica's mom that much *better* than me?

Mother's Day is a form of torture. Even the "creator" of Mother's Day, Anna Jarvis, turned against it within a decade. Being forced to "show" your appreciation for your mom on a single day of the year doesn't work for most kids, or for moms. (Or for Dad's who have one day to orchestrate a love fest that will sustain their wives through another year of parenting.) I prefer my "appreciation" in smaller, more regular doses.

One good thing about Mother's Day is that it gives me a chance to think about how well I'm doing as a parent. I get to give myself an honest "annual review." What am I really teaching my kids versus what I think I am teaching them? I'm a role model, like it or not. Am I a good one? Good or bad, they are learning their future parenting skills from me. This is worth thinking about. Especially if I want grandchildren I can tolerate.

Luckily I have children who aren't shy about telling me what I'm doing wrong.

My youngest claims she is writing a parenting book based on her experiences as my daughter. Every time I mess up, my daughter says something like, "That's going to be Chapter 4, on how *not* to inspire your daughter to do better in math ..." It's her way of pointing out my "bad parenting" moments in a lighthearted, non-threatening way. Surely she wouldn't actually publish a "tell-all" book exposing my mommy-dearest moments? Actually, she might. This keeps me on my toes. Clever girl. I hope she learned this "art of war" approach from me.

I know very well that I am not perfect. And it's not just because my kids tell me so. I most often fail by being too busy. With work and three kids, I don't always manage to attain parenting "best practices." On the positive side, running my own business allows me to make my own hours. I have the flexibility to go to their school concerts and stay home with them when they are sick. On the negative side, I get to make my own hours. So I work *all* the time. To quote another of my kids' Mother's Day poems, "Click Click Click, hear the sound of Mommy's mouse, Click Click Click." Yeah, I get the message.

That said, I firmly believe that my working benefits my daughters. I know that my girls respect the fact that I run a business *and* that I'm a mom. They see how I've managed work and motherhood, and while it's not easy, they know it can be done. I learned the same lesson from my own working mother. So, while I often screw up and forget to pick up a kid (and sometimes other peoples' kids), the psychological damage to my children does not seem permanent. My girls have ambition, but unlike me at a young age, they are also sure they want to have kids. They are much more balanced than I ever was.

Just a few weeks ago, my daughter came back from a play date and told me that she wouldn't trade me for any other mommy she knows. I was very happy. I think it's because I let her eat a half bag of marshmallows – an unintended consequence of not paying enough attention. But I have to believe that her desire to be my child runs a little deeper than marshmallow consumption. (Or maybe I should find out what happened at that play date. Something made her realize that I wasn't so bad after all.)

I'd like to think she wants to be with me versus the family with the mansion and the indoor swimming pool because she recognizes my inner awesomeness. She and I might even share some core values and interests, as well as genes. I know she respects that I work hard, because when she's showing a new friend around the house, she describes my office as the place where "my mom runs a big business."

In the end, I think she sticks with me because she knows that eight out of ten times, I put her first. If she *really* needs me, I will be there. Moms are, after all, forever.

When work threatens, my Mother's Day cards help put me back on the right path. My "flower" card is taped next to my computer. I'm smart enough to know that the mom so lovingly described in this card is not me. She is a Platonic Ideal. I will never be that perfect. But the fact that "she" exists, if only in my daughters' minds, reminds me to quit for the day and go spend some time with my kids.

While they still want me around.

# PART THREE

# I'M NO SUPERWOMAN

ભ ભ ભ

*Women, regardless of how they have chosen to lead their lives, can now breathe a sigh of relief that superwoman is dead.*

– Deborah J. Swiss

# No Longer Green with Envy over the Red Book

*Holly Madden*

When "it" arrived five years after college, I read through it with youthful curiosity. When it showed up ten years after college, I received it with dread, but read it anyway. When it was delivered yet again fifteen years after college, I didn't even break the seal. I left it in its plastic packaging and tossed it in a closet along with some old, faded gym shorts from the '80s.

"It" is the red-covered Harvard class report that is sent out to alumni every five years. It is a compilation of missives submitted by my former classmates that describe their latest career and personal accomplishments. It is thick. It is intimidating. It can make you feel like an utter failure after reading just two pages.

When the latest edition of the *Red Book* arrived this past spring, something strange happened. I opened it up as soon as I got it, pored through the pages, smiled, even laughed. After closing it, I was even happier. Because I realized, for the first time in the twenty years since graduation, I no longer lived in fear of the *Red Book*.

To understand why, let's back up a little. When I was growing up, my mom always held up the careers of others to inspire my own. She was Old School. She admired lawyers, doctors, and professors. If you chose one of those professions, you were sure to be well-respected in society, live in a big house, and have lots of dough so you'd never have to worry. I understand why she felt this way. She was one of three children raised in the wake of the Great Depression and her family always worried about being able to pay their bills.

After she became a mom, she scrimped, saved and did everything possible to position me for success in life. And her definition of success was becoming a lawyer, doctor, or professor. The problem was, as much I tried to ignore it, my creative side was stronger and louder than my lawyerly side. And much to my parents' dismay, I went into the creative side of the advertising field. Mind you: I did so knowing full well that my Harvard education did not prepare me in the least bit for this career path.

In the years that followed, I paid my dues. My Ivy League degree may have helped get me job interviews, but it certainly didn't give me any fast track to the top. One rung at a time, I worked my way up from secretary to junior copywriter to senior copywriter to creative director. There were small, gratifying successes along the way, but no major event that, for my parents, would offset my failure to take on the coveted role of doctor or lawyer. I was fairly happy in my life and what I was doing, but I couldn't jettison the feeling that I wasn't living up to my Harvard grad potential. And when that big fat red class report arrived every five years, it only served to underscore my feelings of career underachievement.

When I paged through the thick booklet, it was so easy to feel intimidated. Heck, there was the gal who played hockey with my former college roommate who was now a major TV network producer. There was that seemingly dopey lacrosse player (whom I sort of dated) who became a well-respected physician. There was that guy who used to hold the three-day keg parties who now headed up a division at one of New York's most prominent investment banking firms.

And there was me. Married. Advertising Professional. Ho Hum Holly. Of course, I was happy for my former classmates and their successes. But I'll be honest: reading about them made me feel extremely defeated. Why couldn't I have made something of my Harvard degree to the level they had? Was I not motivated enough? Was I not smart enough? Was I not something else enough?

These were the gnawing questions that plagued me every time that #%& class report showed up on my doorstep. And these are the questions I finally stopped asking when, in 2001, I became a mom.

Once in the throes of Motherhood, there was no time for self-assessment. There was only time for doing. I was lucky to have a few minutes to suck down a triple espresso and wipe the gobs of spit-up out of my hair. My benchmark for success wasn't lowered, but it did change. Getting my son to not pee on my shirt when I changed his diaper? Major victory. Convincing my son not to throw his bottle on the floor of the car and burst into tears about it? Huge breakthrough. Several bleary-eyed months passed by and then one day it hit me: All that stuff I used to worry about? It didn't matter anymore. There was no more wondering what I should be doing in life. This was it. No other "job" I had before had tested me so fiercely or rewarded me so richly. After a lifetime of searching, I had found the role I was always meant to play.

So, when *Red Book* time rolled around again (this time for my twentieth class reunion), I did something different. When I got the form from Harvard asking me to submit a missive for the upcoming Class Book, I didn't scoff at it and say aloud, "What do I have to promote?" I actually sat down and wrote a missive about myself and my new role as a mom. Sure, in some people's eyes it wasn't nearly impressive as the guy who became a professor at a prominent law school; or the woman who is now the editor of a major metropolitan newspaper; or the many other former classmates who have conquered, discovered, invented, prevailed, or pioneered. But in my mind, it conveyed a success story nonetheless.

And when that *Red Book* did arrive, I picked it up and read it enthusiastically. Perhaps the best part was reading missives that sounded a lot more genuine than they had in the past. Instead of bragging about their career achievements, more of my former classmates shared their personal, and refreshingly honest, stories of triumph and failure. There were battles with cancer. There were jobs lost and marriages that fell apart. There were heart-breaking stories of people who went through unimaginable things. And then there was the missive of a guy, a father, who counted among his blessings:

"Proud papa of bar mitzvah; incurable idealist; inventor of the Hug of a Thousand Kisses; thinking about resuming meditation."

It turns out that, as we Harvard alums grow older, we're becoming more real, more honest, more aware of what success can and should mean. And because we are, the *Red Book* has become a more interesting read than ever before. Who would have thought?

# WILL THE REAL MOTHERS PLEASE STAND UP?

*Alaina Sheer*

L et's get the record straight, shall we?
I'm a mom, not a superhero.

Superheroes, by definition, have powers that are super human –
like leaping tall buildings in a single bound, wielding magic lassos,
casting storm clouds, or even breathing under water. Last week, on
Twitter, a father I know sent me a message from the war zone: "I'm
@ home all day with sick baby (wife's outta town). Don't know how
you do this all the time by yourself. You are superhuman."

I smiled and wrote back, "I know. Crazy, isn't it? CRAZY. And
that is why I tell people I am allowed to lose it every once in a while.
Thanks for the props."

I hear it in the most genuine of ways from married parents whose
spouse leaves town for the weekend. But last I checked, my only
"super powers" are being able to clean the kitchen and entertain my
son at the same time, change a dirty diaper without gagging, and
grocery shop without losing my mind. I may be a single working
mother, but all moms, single or not, are not "super" anything. We
are just human. And some of us, like me, may need more help than
others. We adapt in any given environment because we have to – it's
motherhood, baby.

During my pregnancy, as every mother I know has done, I
worked full-time. On the Friday before my due date, two days after
the event I'd been planning for the last three months had gone off

without a hitch, I sat down for dinner and my water broke. I was ready.

Three months earlier, starting to swell and so incredibly tired, I remember asking myself, "What am I going to do when he actually gets here? How do women do this? How will I work (successfully) and raise a child?"

There were no clear answers. Every book, every magazine, every movie and TV show had painted pictures of these superhero moms doing it all without breaking a sweat. These mythical creatures, like Mrs. Brady and Mrs. Cleaver, are buried in our psyches. If we are not the perfect mother with sparkling white toilets and fresh cookies every Sunday, we are failures.

Then something amazing happened. I discovered an article in *Elle* magazine by Gloria Steinem entitled, "Success is not doing it all."

"It's impossible," she wrote, "for women to do it all." By telling us that a successful woman should work full-time, be a mother, a wife and, let's not forget, look fabulous doing it, society is actually setting us up to feel like failures. To quote Steinem, this idea of doing it all is actually the "enemy of equality, not the path to it."

Here's the part of the article that burned into my mind when I read it: "The women's rights movement isn't finished."

The pressure of motherhood in today's world is unbelievable, and it comes at us from every direction, every day, every hour, and every minute. If we're doing one thing, we're often thinking about another. If we're working, we wish we could be home with the kids. If we're staying at home, we wonder what it would be like to have that career. But while raising a human is arguably the most important job on this planet, there are no exceptional clauses to protect mothers in the work place. For example, we can't leave work early to pick up our children from school – no parent can without putting their job in jeopardy.

I tore the article out and stuck it to my office wall so I could read it every day during my pregnancy. Somehow, her words had enlightened me to the fact that I had to write a new definition for success – my own definition.

Today, with the advent of blogs and all other forms of online communication, millions of moms are rewriting the definition of success by telling their own stories. The real stories from the trenches of motherhood have emerged.

Many women's magazine and television websites allow you to leave comments to offer up your opinion. The collective voice we hear is no longer being dictated to us, but being written by us. And this is just the beginning. (You can't see my face or hear my voice right now, but I'm beaming with excitement I'm an eternal optimist when it comes to the human spirit, especially the spirits of women).

As a mommy blogger, I have been one of many voices in the community of single mothers for over a year now. Finding my voice and connecting with other women like me has saved my sanity and pulled me through my darkest moments. Now, when I pick up a magazine bursting with supermodels and extravagantly expensive handbags, I find myself staring at strangers – impersonators – with hollow faces and unstained shirts. Then I toss the magazine in the trash and open up my laptop to find real mothers, real women.

Their voices whisper in my head throughout my day. If another mother tells me she understands my pain and has her own, I feel less alone. As mothers, we think, we create, and we make mistakes. We realize that we are not superheroes, never were, and never wanted to be.

# FEMINIST MOTHERHOOD ... SAY WHAT?

*Michelle Levine*

Feminist. Motherhood. How's that for a mouthful? I had no idea the two went together until I became a mother. And then it all started falling into place. The slow and painful realization that there is no turning back; no one told you it would be this way, and no, none of it is fair.

I usually don't even know what day of the week it is, but I can remember exactly where I was six years ago when I realized I had "gender issues." That was the phrase I settled on because I certainly did not identify myself as a feminist. The word just has such a negative connotation. I'm a child of the '70s, and I remember hearing about the ERA and bra burning and Gloria Steinem, but not in a positive way. Besides, it wasn't sexy to be a feminist. The lady on the perfume commercial, she was sexy. Sure, her catchy jingle might have been an empowering little tune about doing it all, but the visuals had nothing to do with that message. As I recall, she was done up in a clingy wrap dress, wearing heels and striking seductive poses as she pouted and sang, "I can bring home the bacon/Fry it up in a pan/And never ever let you forget you're a man/'Cause I'm a woman." Brilliant, right?

And this was aimed toward ... whom, exactly? The housewife who wanted to get a job and might entertain the notion that wearing the advertised perfume would magically bestow her with the ability to happily work outside the home all day, return home to cook a nourishing dinner for her family and spend the evening as her husband's love slave? Or was it more of a reassuring message for men? Don't worry, guys. The girls have been acting a little crazy lately, but it'll all work out. Women can earn some money outside the home and still cook for and cater to you, all the while looking fabulous and smelling good.

Funny, the jingle said nothing about kids. And that's the punch line society delivers too late. You can have it all and do it all … just not if you want to be a mom. You've come a long way, baby … until you have a baby. That reality was never mentioned in the "you can be anything you want to be when you grow up, honey" pep talks my generation received as little girls. Instead, we were raised with the belief that it was our birthright – indeed, our obligation – to pursue a career, to honor the courageous women who fought for our right to work and have choices.

So it came as a bit of a shock to find myself on maternity leave feeling like I had no choices. Where had I gone wrong? I was a good girl in high school, graduated as salutatorian, went to an Ivy League college, came to the big city to study and practice law, and even had the good fortune to meet my handsome husband along the way and be blessed with a precious son. I had crossed the finish line, hadn't I? So where were the cape and the superpowers I had been promised? Hell, where was that bottle of perfume and the frying pan?

I wasn't feeling very empowered. I was feeling tricked and misled and angry. Why had I worked my ass off to start a career that I would only have to derail once I gave birth? Because I could? Because I needed a JD on the wall above the changing table? And wasn't that the same JD my husband had, from the same school? But he earned more, and I was, after all, the mother, so it was time to embark on the endlessly entertaining merry-go-round of "I can't afford to stay home, so I will continue working, but childcare is so expensive that I am really just working to pay the daycare center so why am I working at all especially when I am a mother now and aren't mothers supposed to be home raising their own babies?" Were these the choices I was supposed to be grateful for?

And so it was that a child was born … and right behind him, a feminist mother.

*Originally published on Mothers Movement Online.*

# You'll Never Look Like Heidi Klum

*Heather Cabot*

Heidi Klum burst my bubble this week. *The Project Runway* host, Victoria's Secret model and mother of four, mercilessly threw cold water on my fantasy that, with enough will power and working out, my postpartum body could one day resemble hers. In an interview with *Marie Claire* magazine, she said, "You can't kid yourself; you couldn't bounce back to being model slim post-baby if you didn't start off like that to begin with." Really? Yup, it's true.

Seriously, I do appreciate her candor. The fact is, it's hard not to feel a little deficient when one doesn't emerge from pregnancy looking like she's ready to strut down the catwalk in skimpy lingerie. But with the celebrity baby-bump obsession running at full throttle these days, few new-ish moms can resist aspiring (no matter how unrealistically) to look like preening Hollywood goddesses when they walk out of the hospital.

So, with Heidi in mind, here's a little pep talk for my peeps — those women who are healthy and strong and still don't wear a designer sample size … Let it go! All of this pressure to be perfect takes a lot of the joy out of this new phase of our lives. Frankly, it's not just the happy moments we're missing while we pore over tabloids promising to reveal the post-baby diet secrets of the likes of Christina Aguilera and Denise Richards. All this focus takes a heck of a lot of energy — energy we need just to make it through a typical day of mothering.

I'm not saying this is easy to do. You can't walk into the supermarket without all of those headlines screaming at you about who in Tinseltown is thin or fat these days. And let's be honest; it is a guilty pleasure to kick back and page through the photos (Stars ... They're just like us. Not!) But fun aside, we can try to be a bit more mindful of setting realistic goals and turning our attention to what's really important – being healthy and centered for our families. Letting go of perfection (or the tabloids' image of perfection) can really go a long way.

Of course, the push for perfection transcends fitness and body image. There are women who believe they have to put a hot, home-cooked meal on the table every night ... or women who feel that unless they make partner and manage to get to toddler class once a week, they are "bad mothers." We all have our hang-ups about what it means to be super mom. But we moms need to take stock of what is really important and learn to go a little bit easier on ourselves. One of my favorite new mottos for motherhood is: "Accept imperfection, perhaps even revel in it."

In my own life, I'm trying to embrace this hard lesson. In my quest to stay disciplined and fit while taking care of my twin two-year-olds, running my weekly e-zine, *The Well Mom*, and serving as a consumer spokesperson for Yahoo! (oh, and writing a weekly blog), I decided to train for a triathlon. I even wrote about it in my blog a few months ago. I had the best of intentions. What I failed to realize when I signed up for a training group is that I did not have the time to commit to the coach's program. I was able to modify the workouts to fit my fragmented schedule. But because of family commitments, I just couldn't make it to practice twice a week. Nor did I ever find time to get my bike in shape; learn how to change a flat tire or research renting a wetsuit. Suddenly, this triathlon was starting to add a lot of stress to my life when it was really meant to be something fun. So, after yet another week of missing practice and a run-through with my teammates, I decided this was just not my time to do this particular race. There will be others later this summer and fall ... and later in my life. I feel a weight lifting off my shoulders as I write this!

Heidi Klum is not the first glamorous star to openly discuss the impact of her image on us regular moms. Not too long ago, Julia Roberts chalked up her enviable post-baby figure to genetics (and exercise). We might not like to hear the truth. But kudos to them for telling it like it is and in a sense, setting us free.

I really do believe that beauty comes from within. But when you've spent half the night at the bedside of a sick child, can't remember the last time you bought (or wore) mascara and, despite all of your education, you find yourself unable to complete a sentence by 8 p.m., it's no wonder even super moms lose their inner glow. Yes, those celebrity moms make it look easy with their entourage of trainers, stylists, make-up artists and the like. Moms in the real world know it's a scramble to get out of the house some mornings without breakfast smeared on your sleeve.

That's not making excuses. It's realism.

*Originally published on The Huffington Post, May 2008.*

# FROM HARVARD TO HOMEMAKING

*Bracha Goetz*

From Harvard to.... homemaking? It was not a big jump down, as most people assume.

After graduating from Harvard University at the top of my department in 1977, I went on to medical school, responding seemingly well to the intense "nouveau" pressure for young women like me to succeed professionally. But during my first year in medical school, I started to panic. It felt as if only my outer self was moving ahead, leaving the most intrinsic, characteristic parts of me behind. It was as if I was starting to remember the way I used to be before the societal influences shifted dramatically.

Couldn't I still have a choice? Couldn't I choose not to become a professional career woman? What if I were to actually work up the nerve to do something extremely embarrassing like devote my intelligence and creative abilities to building a good marriage and trying to raise my own children in an exemplary home? Was that option still available, even though I never heard it mentioned anymore? The more I let myself wonder about it freely, the more I knew it was what I most wanted even if everyone else at that time thought I had flipped my lid.

Today people no longer think that I'm nuts. Today the value of my choice is clearly evident. Not in shining glassware or sparkling clean floors like a stereotypic '50s homemaker might have squealed about. It is evident in the shining character traits of six children, now grown big, and in the extra sparkle that's in their eyes.

Through the years, many people have asked me how a Harvard grad, a woman who loves to think, could become a homemaker. I feel that in order to be devoted to being a homemaker, a mother, and a guide to trusting souls, a woman has to love to think. Being a homemaker, with an awareness of the potential inherent in the position, is the most challenging intellectual pursuit I could ever envision.

I cannot possibly counterbalance the many influences that devalue homemaking by considering it a mindless endeavor that anyone can do. Hopefully, I can still open up a few minds to the fact that in order to do a great job as a homemaker, we really have to make great use of our most prized mental capabilities. After all, homemaking is far from simple or mindless.

In marriage and in parenting, we are given the opportunity to create something far, far more beautiful than a Rembrandt masterpiece. We have the chance to help create a real live masterpiece of a human being. A gigantic amount of thinking is required in order to shape and mold fine character traits. Even though some people are born with easier dispositions to work with than others, there is so much room for growth in every person. Each individual holds many hidden treasures. And in digging for them, we invariably end up uncovering some of our own.

It takes much time and thought to guide children to become truly good people. And it is still possible in this day and age to raise pure, appreciative, joyful children. The thing is, it requires a lot of brain power to override the abundant influences working against achieving this goal. We need to understand well who each constantly evolving individual child is in order to be able to guide him or her along the unique pathway that can lead to the fulfillment of his or her highest potential.

What kind of intellectual skills are needed in order to strive toward greatness in parenting? There are the finely tuned skills needed to assess whether or not a child is capable of moving on to his or her own next stage of development. There are the perceptual powers required in order to determine the best time to step forward and help out a child, or step back and let the child try to work out a problem on his own, without our involvement. And there are cognitive abilities that are a prerequisite for teaching children the skills that will enable them to make themselves happy in life. These are the skills that enable children to transform negative experiences into positive ones, work through angry emotions, and learn to appreciate all that they have.

There is a tremendous amount of pre-planning that goes into good parenting, and there is also plenty of on-the-spot quick thinking needed, too. Parents have to figure out the most effective ways to help their children understand how to get along with others, how to circumvent fights, and how to feel confident being themselves. Parents also need to study well and know when to implement the systematic skills that help minimize whining, tantrums and disrespectful behavior.

Everyone readily admits that parenting is physically and emotionally demanding. But, intellectually demanding? That's overlooked. The ironic part is that parenting would be dramatically less demanding physically and emotionally if more of our intellectual abilities were utilized in the process.

Then, there are the people who tell me that with today's economy the way it is, it is no longer a viable option for women to be home with their children. I'm here to prove that it is still a wonderful choice readily available, especially for women with intellectual prowess. We live simply, but with a much higher quality of life than most harried families, who are always rushing about with no time to enjoy what they're hurrying after. Our children have an enthusiastic appreciation for even the smallest of things. And that, I believe, is one of the most valuable gifts a parent can ever receive.

A synthesis of values from the homebound '50s, freeing '60s and '70s, and overextended '80s, '90s and '00s can now, hopefully, begin to culminate into a much deeper and broader view, encompassing all the options from which a woman can honestly choose.

As women come to respect parenting more, making their theoretical priorities a reality, they can devote more of their talents and concentration to their children. When we help our children grow up beautifully, we will at the same time be helping ourselves to grow in the most authentic way possible.

We can still have fulfilling marriages. We can still have respectful, responsible children involved with us in a mutually rewarding relationship. But too many minds still remain shut to the intellectually stimulating potential of homemaking. Well, they always told me that my Harvard education would open doors. These are the closed doors I hope to open.

*Originally published in The Jewish Press, October 2008.*

# IS THIS THE AMERICAN DREAM?

*Kezia Willingham*

I t's early September – latent summer in Seattle. When I leave for work in the morning, it is cool enough for a light jacket. I know that on the commute home I will be sweating. My thirteen-month-old son clings to me as I give him a hug at the front door. The precise second when the curl of his lip begins to turn from smile to frown crushes me. I pry him from my arms, handing him to my husband.

When I became a mother, I was young, single and on welfare. My choice was never "to work or not to work," it was what type of job I could get. I wanted more for my child than to scrape by on minimum wage, so I went back to school, earning both bachelor's and master's degrees. At one point, I dreamed of becoming a policy maker in D.C. Another time, I hoped to become a college professor. As a poor, single mom, I had to reign in these dreams to pursue the reality of a living wage. My first job out of school was with the local school system, which allowed me to have time with my daughter while meeting the conditions I required of work – paid vacations, sick leave, and health benefits.

In pursuit of the American Dream, I fell in love and got married; eventually, my husband and I purchased our first house, a symbol of stability and success. For us, it also meant an end to housing assistance, inspections, and neighbors whose screams filtered through the floors and walls of cheaply constructed apartments. My new job for Seattle Head Start would ensure that children enrolled in the program receive the annual medical exams mandated by the state. I liked my job. I had my own cubicle, where I hung photos of my family. I had access to office supplies and a great view of the industrial south side of the city – the port, Amtrak, graffitied walls.

Our American Dream came to a crashing halt when we received a call from my husband's immigration attorney, informing us that his Adjustment of Status application had been denied by the Department of Homeland Security. His work permit had been terminated due to a crime he had committed five years earlier. If we were to appeal the decision, it could take as long as two years for the paperwork to be processed and cost at least $10,000 more than the $10,000 we'd already placed on his credit cards for the application that had been denied. We were in the process of closing on a $300,000 home, I had $70,000 in student-loan debt, and my husband was still paying off his last attempt to try to become a permanent resident of this country. We simply couldn't afford to fight the charges.

I didn't know my husband when he committed the crime. It was crime of passion, as they say in the movies. He had gone to see the mother of his son, a woman with whom he was deeply in love. When he found her with another man, he lost control. He raced through the apartment, threatened the man with a kitchen knife, and wrestled him to the floor. Nobody was hurt. By the time the police arrived, both men were gone.

My husband turned himself in the next day and paid $5,000 to a lawyer who convinced him to plead guilty to felony counts of domestic violence and residential burglary. He served six months in jail before being released for good behavior. He entered a year-long, court-ordered treatment group for domestic violence, paid his fines and found a new job, which he held until the termination of his work permit.

I've thought often about the crime my husband committed, about how one bad decision can permanently affect the rest of your life. I've hated my husband for being so foolish, and I've hated the immigration system for being so unforgiving. When I am not resentful, I understand how helpless he must have felt, watching his family disintegrate in the embrace of another man. I see how important family is to him, how he would do anything for us, like assuming the role of caretaker when I go to work. For a working class Latino man, this is no small concession. I imagine how the pain and fear of losing his family erupted in a flash, destroying all rational thought and resulting in consequences far greater than he was able to conceive at the time.

It's been close to a year since I have become the breadwinner in our family. On paper, I make more than I ever have before. I am a homeowner. On the outside, it would appear that I "have it all." In reality, the mortgage takes up 85% of my net earnings. There is not enough left to feed my family. My husband will most likely be deported. Panic and anxiety are as much a part of my daily functioning as breath. I've never felt quite as hopeless as I do now.

As I drive toward my office, I pass homeless women and men of all different colors, some weaving through the streets inebriated, some clad in tight jeans and heels, looking to earn a buck, others posted adjacent to on-ramps with cardboard signs asking for help. There was a time in my life when I feared homelessness. So far, I have managed to keep a roof over our heads, but the prospect of losing our house is real.

I visited the food bank for the first time the other day with my children. An hour after we checked in, I slowly walked down the line, pointing to the two cans from each shelf that I wanted. Some people complained loudly about food being past its prime. I gladly accepted what we were given, went home, and prepared a meal.

# MULTIPLE IDENTITY CRISIS

*Berta Davis*

The 1970s were quite magical. Women were meeting in each others' homes, marching in the streets, and discussing what feminism meant to us personally and as a generation. We were college educated and ready to trade in our aprons for a seat in the boardroom. We had lofty goals and believed that with ease and fluidity, without harm to self or family, we could do it all. We never thought of ourselves as "superwomen." It was just what we needed and wanted to do.

For thirty-two years, I have personally and professionally struggled with the challenges of being a working mom. As I look back, I am struck by the difficulties that women, including myself, continue to face. Women today are suffering from what I call a "multiple identity crisis" – by trying to blend the many roles they are supposed to play, they are putting unsustainable demands on themselves and their families. As a therapist, I listen over and over to female clients who berate themselves for not being good enough in any of their given roles: professionals from 9 to 5, mothers 24/7, and lovers whenever they can find the time and energy. I want to apologize to these women and tell them that it is my generation they have to thank for this craziness. We created this model and it just isn't fair!

I am a member of a group of psychologists – seven women who have met monthly for over twenty years. We are friends, colleagues, and mothers, all married or once married. The group was formed to connect with others who shared a commitment to psychology and to advance similar values that we all held dear. As psychologists, we bring not only our own struggles and achievements to the table, but an understanding of how other women are involved in a similar juggling act. In our fifties, sixties and seventies, we have the joy of looking back, as well as the anticipation of looking forward. As the seven of us reminisce about these years, many of us wish we had given ourselves more time to enjoy the delights of being a young mother. We were so worried about losing our professional momentum that we took little time off to enjoy our children. There were economic reasons why many of us worked, but much of our stamina arose from the belief system that we were women of a new age – we were "liberated" – and that it was our duty to do meaningful work outside the home. We didn't focus on what we were missing when we ran off to work at 8 a.m., and we weren't there to help our kids after school. My son ended up going to Princeton, so it couldn't have been that detrimental to him that I wasn't always there. Of course, we felt a pang of sadness when we heard news of the baby's first step or first word from the babysitter, but we comforted ourselves by believing it was in our best interest – women's best interest – to work.

My son was born on a military base in Japan. On the night I went into labor, I decided to teach the class I was scheduled to teach, through labor pains and all, while my husband waited outside in case I needed to go to the hospital. As I look back, I question why I didn't take time off from my work to nurture myself and delight in my newborn son. Like many women of today, I felt that I had something to prove, that I could do it all. Having a baby wasn't going to stop me. I could make it as a mom, a career woman, and a wife.

Recently someone commented on my success in achieving so many of my own life goals. How had I done it? this woman asked. The question was a surprise. I feel that I have been living life on a tightrope, suspended high above the ground, and, more often than not, way off balance. If it appears that I have walked this tightrope with ease and tranquility, then it is an illusion. Balancing the roles of wife, mother and professional has never been easy for me. I have worked hard, tried to accept my failures with as much grace as possible, celebrated my successes as they have come, and all the while continued to learn – and accept – that I can't do it all.

I'm no superwoman, after all. Is anybody?

# A LETTER TO THE NEXT GENERATION

*Karen Sibert*

It's an unpopular view, but no, young ladies, you really can't do it all. In the heady days of the 1970s and '80s, women came to believe that all a girl needed was determination enough and she could be and do anything she ever wanted. I'm here to tell you that there's more to the story.

As an anesthesiologist, my colleagues – both doctors and nurses – often ask me to take care of them and their families when they need anesthesia, and surgeons request me for challenging cases. The orchid on my kitchen windowsill was a gift from a grateful patient, and I'm lucky enough to love what I do. My husband also practices anesthesiology, and he understands better than anyone that some days I get home late because I can't leave until surgery ends and my patient is safely tucked into the recovery room. I'm a mom, too – not a soccer mom or a hockey mom – but nonetheless, a mother of three. My older daughter has a master's degree, a good job, and a wonderful husband. My son is a pre-med sophomore in college, and my younger daughter just left to start her freshman year.

So where's the downside? As a woman, you can juggle many things fairly well, but you will never be the perfect wife and mother and have a high-powered career at the same time. There aren't enough hours in the day or enough brain cells in your head. Marriage? I've been divorced, and my husband deserves a lot more of my attention than he usually gets. It's lucky that he can cook. The children? They learned early that if they forgot lunch in the morning, no one was going to hop in a minivan and bring it to school. No doubt there were a thousand lapses in my mothering that they still resent, although I did read them a lot of bedtime stories. They have borne up for the most part with cheer and fortitude – and thankfulness that they weren't burdened, like some of their friends, with "helicopter moms" who hovered constantly and watched their every move.

My career? I started medical school in 1979, four years after my first child was born, and I have worked full-time ever since. Some procedures in anesthesia require technical skills that I would quickly lose if I performed them less often. However, I am not a department chairman in a medical school, or a researcher on the cutting edge of medical discovery. Because I have a family, I've downscaled some of my ambitions. My group practice is large and enables me to take time off when it's important. Once I'm done for the day and leave the hospital, unless I'm on call, my pager is off. Over time I have come to terms with what men have known all along: you can't be a CEO or the president of the United States or even a hardworking wage-earner and still make it to all the soccer games, or be the room mother who brings healthy snacks to school. You won't always be around to give a reassuring hug at the exact moment a child needs one. Something has to give. Once you acknowledge that you can't do it all, you can figure out where you need to be when it really matters.

Recently a surgeon approached me and said, "Are you here on Thursday? I need you; I have a patient for an esophagogastrectomy." I replied, "Sorry, no. My son is having his tonsils out." My son isn't a baby; he's nineteen years old and would have been perfectly able to get a friend to give him a ride to the surgery center. That wasn't the point. The point is that the patient undergoing a major operation deserved to have an anesthesiologist who was fully engaged in taking care of him. My mind would have been elsewhere. So we arranged for another anesthesiologist to take care of the patient, and I took the day off to be with my son. He seemed pleased to have me there.

My thirty-three years as a mother lead me to conclude that some jobs are too important to multi-task. My patients can count on the fact that when I'm at work, my full attention is with them, and the rest of the time – well, I do my best, and luckily I never set my sights on the award for "Mother of the Year."

*Originally published in the Journal of the California Society of Anesthesiologists, 2008*

# PART FOUR

# DIVIDED LIVES

ରେଷେରେ

*When I was at work..., I always felt like I was shortchanging my girls. But then when I was at home, I was worried that I was letting people at work down.*

– Michelle Obama

# MUTHERING HEIGHTS

*Alexandra Bradner*

*[T]oday's moms could well be facing "demands that are historically unprecedented," says Sharon Hays, a sociologist at the University of Virginia and author of* The Cultural Contradictions of Motherhood. *"Their world is child-centered, expert-guided, emotionally intense and financially expensive."*

> – Marco R. della Cava, "The Bands that Rock the Cradle," 1/31/05, *USA Today*.

I don't even like *USA Today*, but this article – about mothers who moonlight in punk rock bands – stuck with me. Only two days into my new position as a philosophy professor at a small, Midwestern, liberal arts college, I found myself complaining to my older male colleagues at lunch that GenX parenting was "child-centered, expert-guided, emotionally intense, and financially expensive." Not a terrific career move. I was just so overwhelmed and preoccupied by the tension between my two lives that I couldn't keep my mouth shut.

The past few years have delivered a move to Appalachia, a house purchase, a pregnancy, a baby, a year of nursing, a dissertation defense, a house sale, another house purchase, a move to the Midwest, a new job, a miscarriage, the death of my father, a third pregnancy, gestational diabetes, a second baby, another year of nursing, two infant asthma attacks, and a mid-tenure review. To make matters even more interesting, I've spent much of this time single parenting, as my partner of eighteen years endures half of each week at his own academic post three hours away. So while I'm usually more of a Spoon-Raconteurs fan, as I drive to work these days, I find myself lingering on the heavy metal stations. In *Wuthering Heights*, Catherine Earnshaw's divided attention drove her mad. I don't think I'm there just yet, but I'm pretty irritated.

People certainly make many of their own choices, and clearly, women of my income and education have more control over their lives than most. But I can't help but wonder how many times we have to hear that the American Academy of Pediatrics recommends a year of breastfeeding and that the most important years of cognitive development are between zero and three before we enact more humane maternity policies in the workplace. Children need their mothers – not nannies or daycare workers – to narrate the mundane, introduce so many joys, and assist with so many pains. Only someone in love with a child can get down on the floor around the fourth hour of care and invest in a puzzle. So we should be at home. But women need a public voice, external affirmation, internal feelings of triumph, money of their own, and a mental life beyond worry and logistics. Only those free to fulfill their early promise have a chance of living through their fifties and sixties without debilitating regret. So we should be able to work as well.

> *If we don't salt the walkway, the postal carrier is going to slip • Someone has to be home at 10 a.m., so the contractor can show us the tile • They didn't have narrow ballet slippers, so we have to go back to pick up a special order • The amoxicillin will be ready at 3 p.m. • When I picked up Martha Nussbaum at the airport, there was a dirty diaper in the car—Martha Nussbaum! • We need more two-percent organic milk, applesauce, and coffee Häagen Dasz.*

My three year old, Vivian, has just moved from puzzles and stand-alone toys to play sets and pretend play. She is quite into Nanny McPhee, a sweet British film starring Emma Thompson, and takes great pleasure in acting out the various scenes. One day, she was running around the house pretending to be Simon, the mischievous ringleader of a band of sibling terrors. So I thought I'd join in the fun and encourage creative play by acting out the scene with special objects only a good mother could appropriate and re-imagine. In this particular vignette, the kids put baby Aggie in a pot of wet greens on the kitchen table; so I brought down a pot, put a doll inside of it, and waited happily in the kitchen for her to come running. Well, she ran in, took one look at her mom with a baby in a cooking pot, and started to cry, mumbling between streaming tears, "Mommies don't cook babies. Mommies don't cook babies." That's right. My daughter now thinks it's in the realm of possibility that I might cook her.

> *Please write a check for the bowling field trip before you leave • We could take the whole pile to that shred-it for charity event • My family wants to change the Macatawa date to a later weekend • Mir didn't sleep this morning, so she can't go to daycare until 1 p.m. • I'll fix it after I untangle the slinky • The vacuum cleaner doesn't work. • We need more two-percent organic milk, applesauce, and coffee Häagen Dasz.*

Last year, my father was diagnosed with pancreatic cancer. Three months later, he was dead, his inability to process life's sweetness ultimately taking over his body, as well as his mind. By all reports, my dad was never the same after he returned from his second tour in Vietnam, but I never knew why. Already a lawyer, he was commissioned as a military intelligence officer and placed in charge of certifying Viet Cong and North Vietnamese death counts, so his superiors could report casualty rates to the media. Apparently, after refusing to inflate these numbers, he was punished with a reassignment to the darkest zone of the Tet Offensive and never quite recovered from the brutalities he witnessed there. So I was preoccupied for the rest of the day, thinking that it would have been nice to know all of this earlier—a lot earlier. The occasion was complicated by the fact that I was seven months pregnant, managing diabetes and some kind of high clotting marker, and mothering a three-year old. So … what to tell little Vivian (too old to be oblivious and too young to understand) about death and its accompanying cultural practices?

"Mommy, if Poppy was so big, why is the box that Nana is

burying so small?"

Dear, tiny, wide-eyed, innocent child … We set Poppy on fire.

I ended up telling her that when people die, all of the liquid in the body dries up and they shrink. But despite what grownups say to protect their children, they know. And my eldest daughter has remained a peculiarly dark, and somewhat anxious, kid. If grandfathers can die, so can mommies. So can daddies. And so can little children.

*Can you make the lunches and lay out the clothes tonight, so breakfast isn't so crazy? • There were three bathroom trips last night, so good luck getting her up at 7 a.m. • We need to sign up for spring soccer by Saturday morning • It's parent's day at Vivian's ballet class this weekend • Everyone is bringing a homemade dish to the party • We still have three returns left from the holidays • We need more two-percent organic milk, applesauce, and coffee Häagen Dasz.*

Vivian was raised on a modified form of Dr. Sears' attachment parenting. We never left her with a sitter. I nursed instead of pumping. We slept in a family bed. This is all rumored to produce centered, confident, and assured children, because they encounter the world from a place of attachment, calm, and security. And this may eventually turn out to be the case. But it sure is hard for an attached little three-year-old to sit by herself as she watches her mom nurse a newborn all day. Vivian started to pick her lips … off – in other words, until they were bloody. Horror! I was going to have a child who slowly pulled her hair out, obsessively washed her hands, checked each step before putting her weight on it, boiled her combs each night to eliminate bacteria, packed thousands of worthless comics into plasticine envelopes, placed the envelopes into white, acid-free boxes, and, finally, stacked the boxes into bookshelves lining a series of several climate-controlled, storage facilities … I was going to have to raise my father.

So I did what any truly panicked, erstwhile feminist would do. I went out to Toys "R" Us and bought the most desirable object of the Preschool Gaze I could think of—$120 worth of pink, glittery Barbie crap from China. And it worked. By slowly incenting her with the *Barbie in The 12 Dancing Princesses* DVD, the *Barbie & the Diamond Castle* pink, horse-drawn, singing chariot, a genitally ambivalent surfing Ken, several smaller, unfortunate Kelly dolls, and much, much more, we nipped this behavior in the bud. She's now ripping off her fingernails instead. But I'm told this is almost normal.

All was going well until a month ago, when she expressed an interest in Medieval Europe. 'Wow,' I thought. She's advanced! So I rushed to borrow a beautiful library book about medieval feasts, filled with gorgeous pictures and informative text. We sat down to read, and she was delighted by the story in which a lord was preparing to host a visiting King and Queen. Right in the middle of an illustration of the giant kitchen sat a delicacy called "cockatrice," which is half peacock, half deer. "How do they make that?" she asked, wide-eyed (and not in a good way). Well, they slice each animal in half and then sew the different halves together. Luckily, her dad's a vegetarian. So the only disturbing and morally ambiguous person in the house … is me.

> *Miranda was poked in the eye, so we're at the urgent care. Can you call and make an appointment with an ophthalmologist for tomorrow morning?* • *The wiper broke off the front car window, so I just went to Abe's Garage* • *We need more two-percent organic milk, applesauce, and coffee Häagen Dasz.*

In academia, every new semester brings a liberating sense of renewal. Once again, it all seems within reach; everything is possible. But now that I'm approaching forty, it isn't. And who cares, right? Most philosophers of free will agree that freedom from all constraint would be randomness, and that's not what we mean by "freedom" (that's your twenties.) We can't praise or blame random acts. Freedom only really hooks up to responsibility if that freedom is constrained. So the query for the middle-aged mother, who has to raise her children within rules and institutions established and governed by capitalist men, is a truly philosophical puzzle—how to really live within suddenly real constraints. Our professional worlds – replete with late nights, weekends, and the general expectation of ever-readiness – are structured on the assumption that everyone has a stay-at-home wife. Our most demanding work – toward tenure, partner, director, or VP – occurs during the average six years we spend pregnant, breastfeeding, and chasing after toddlers. Most of our fields have no reentry culture.

And that's merely the political. What of the personal? Unlike our mothers, we grew up fully powerful in classroom environments that acknowledged and even celebrated our achievements. We then moved on to jobs and graduate schools in which we succeeded on universal terms. So no wonder we can't adjust to our midlife mediocrity. No longer gunners at work and barely decent mothers, we're damped down, disoriented, and frazzled versions of ourselves. Our quantum state of work-life superposition has led to some practical advance, but conceptually, we're an uncomfortable muddle.

The situation for our children is almost the reverse. Without our attention, without our rules, they live unconstrained in the context of care institutions with 1:6 ratios and names that invariably include words like "learning" and "love." They roam blankly about these toxic-foam-matted rooms, swatting at each other, consuming "health" bars and juices built out of refined sugars and modified starches, looking at garish plastic toys without knowing how to play with them, and waiting for their heavy diapers to be changed. Their energy is unchanneled, their vocabularies underdeveloped, and their cognitive potential untapped. Instead of being frustrated with all the ways in which so many new constraints are chipping away at their identities, they're prevented from forming any true identity but that of the generic company kid. And we stand back, mystified that verbal skills and creativity are on the decline while obesity and school violence are on the rise.

*Apparently, the problem is that Kevin won't return Vivian's hugs •
Your mom called and said she hasn't talked to you or the girls in more
than a week • For her birthday, she wants her friends to dress up as
characters from the Magic Flute • Do you think it would be possible to
move to Utah for a month-long seminar this summer, with the cat? • We
need more two-percent organic milk, applesauce, and coffee Häagen Dasz.*

In chapter 9 of Emily Brontë's *Wuthering Heights*, Catherine famously announces that, while she is in love with the more secure Edgar Linton, she is one with Heathcliff: "My love for Linton is like the foliage in the woods. Time will change it, I'm well aware, as winter changes the trees. My love for Heathcliff resembles the eternal rocks beneath—a source of little visible delight, but necessary … I *am* Heathcliff—he's always, always in my mind, not as a pleasure, any more than I am always a pleasure to myself—but as my own being."

I love philosophy, and I've worked fairly hard to land a position in my field – one with a nice salary and terrific health benefits, in a town with beautiful housing and good schools. But my brooding little Vivian is part of me. And I can't help but think that a society that either forces a mother to choose between her public and private life or ensures she can't succeed when she pursues both, is just tragic and cruel.

*I just sent out the last of the holiday letters • This Saturday is Family Fun Night • Both girls need their vaccination forms signed for the daycare • Who's doing the taxes this year? • One of the other kids said Vivian had a funny name • Our insurance card stopped working at the end of December, so a collection agency called about the nebulizer bill • Miranda ate a piece of cat food • I'm so tired … If you take them for two hours, I'll watch them during the Kentucky game.*

With my spouse gone for half the week and minimal childcare, our house is routinely a wreck, so much so that we're kind of worried about retaining our friends, whom we can never invite over for fear of exposing our squalid living conditions to the community at large. Yesterday, I was down on my hands and knees in a steamy bathroom, scrubbing the tub and wall tile, when Vivian came in to ask a few questions:

"What are you doing?"

"Scrubbing the tub."

"How long is it going to take?"

"Probably about half an hour. I have to do a lot of scrubbing to get the muck off the floor."

"Why do you have to scrub so hard?"

"The muck is really stuck, and I don't want to use any smelly cleaners. So I'm just using some Castile soap, which is a gentle kind of soap and hot water. But it takes a lot of elbow grease."

"What is elbow grease?"

"Well, that means a lot of hard work—a lot of muscle, some patience, focus, imagination, endurance … It's difficult, but I think the extra effort will be worthwhile in the long run."

"Can I sit on your back while you're doing it?"

She hopped on.

> *[And t]he daughter turned out a second edition of the mother …*
>
> – Emily Brontë, *Wuthering Heights*

# QUARTET

*Courtney Cook*

## I

I was nineteen when I became pregnant with my son. It was the spring of my freshman year at Dartmouth. I was not married, nor was I planning to be married. I had not planned to become pregnant. I lived in a dormitory called Richardson, not a three-bedroom house in Winchester, MA, and I was taking Greek and Roman Studies 1 and English 5, not reading through my company's maternity leave policy. My friends were pledging sororities, applying for public service internships, going out three or four nights a week, and studying in the Baker Library stacks on Sunday afternoons. My parents and religious community did not approve of unmarried sex, much less unmarried pregnancy. Still, during the long, frightening summer after my freshman year of college, I decided I wanted to have and raise my baby.

When I returned to Dartmouth the next fall, it was as a married woman, though John – my baby's father and a Dartmouth graduate whose job with the U.S. military was making it possible for me to stay in school – was stationed at Fort Knox, KY. I moved into a dormitory where it was arranged that I could have a room of my own, and I shared a kitchen and a bathroom with four strangers. My friends wanted me to share rooms with them as we had planned to do the previous spring, but I was under the impression that I had to live by myself now that I was married. My professors didn't know I was pregnant. Not even my roommates knew I was pregnant. I didn't want them to. I wore my husband's rugby jerseys and hoped no one would notice. I had a lot of homework that term – my anxiety about staying on track at Dartmouth even though I was about to become a mother drove me to take extra coursework – so I spent most of my time at the library. At home in my tiny bedroom I slept the deep, exhausted sleep of a pregnant, scared college girl. Every so often I walked by myself to the Mary Hitchcock Memorial Hospital obstetrics clinic to hear my baby's heartbeat.

One night, after attending a birthing class in which a midwife stuffed a cabbage patch doll through a foil stove-pipe in order to demonstrate the birthing process, I came home to find my apartment full of people I'd known from the previous year when I'd been just another college freshman – my former roommates, the guys from the floor downstairs, upperclassmen from my freshman year dorm, kids from the campus Christian ministry and my current roommates – having only recently been enlightened as to my "delicate" condition. Somebody had baked a cake in a dormitory kitchen. There were several bottles of Boone's Farm wine. And lots and lots of presents for the baby and me. Copies of *Curious George, Bedtime for Frances, Make Way for Ducklings*, a complete *Winnie the Pooh*, a complete *Adventures of Paddington*, a set of the *Narnia Tales, More, More, More said the Baby, honey I love, One Morning in Maine*, three copies of *Peter Rabbit, The Velveteen Rabbit*, a bunch of books by Richard Scary (the boys brought these, of course), books by Virginia Woolf and T.S. Eliot, books by Beverly Cleary that had been translated into the French *Ramona La Peste*, and *Ramona et son père* and, because it was Dartmouth and he's an alum, a whole lot of Dr. Seuss. There was even a Dr. Seuss book that had been translated into the French, *Yaortu la Tortue (Yurtle, the Turtle)*. Not a single baby outfit, not a play quilt, not a baby food maker, not a playpen, not a breast pump, not a single receiving blanket, not a pair of socks. I was thrilled.

After the term ended, things became a bit more difficult. When I'd finished my last exam, I didn't go home to my family and high school friends in Wyoming as I had the previous year. Instead, I joined John at Fort Knox where the military buildup to the first Persian Gulf War was in full swing. There wasn't any housing on base so we lived in a motel just outside the gates, and there wasn't much for me to do but worry about whether or not John would be sent over. I didn't know any women in the area; my friends were the other twenty-two-year-old Army officers who hung around our motel room with John and me, watching the latest news about the impending ground war and waiting for the baby to be born. I remember how out of place they looked lounging about the maternity ward of Ireland Army Hospital when John Michael Williamson arrived a few weeks later.

We were too inexperienced to appreciate it, but John Michael was a peach of a baby; he took to nursing and sleeping with an aplomb that I now know was exceptional. When he was five weeks' old we loaded up our little Ford Ranger with our few possessions, wedged John Michael's car seat behind the bench, and headed north back up to Dartmouth so that I could resume my studies. On the way there we found out that John's older brother, a husband and father of two and a Navy pilot, had been killed in a military training accident. There was nothing for us to do but continue driving north to Boston and catch a plane back to Oklahoma to John's parents' home. I remember that it was snowing, that the thick wet flakes and the windshield wipers kept an odd sort of time with my husband's tears, and that my baby slept peacefully between feedings the whole way.

A week later, John Michael and I flew back to Boston without John. He couldn't come with us; after his brother's funeral he returned to active army service, this time to Ranger School in far away Fort Benning, Georgia. During a long layover I was so exhausted that I laid my baby right down on the floor of the terminal and curled myself around him. There we both slept until a flight attendant woke me for boarding. On the same flight a business man who must also have been a father cradled John Michael against his clean shirt and tie so I could visit the bathroom. I drove myself home to Hanover through Boston rush hour. The day after we returned was the day I had to register for spring term classes.

I suppose you could say that things settled down after that. I had upgraded my living space from dorm room to motel to a 700-square-foot, unfurnished cinder block apartment in the college's married student housing, and I now owned a crib, a futon, and an old couch scrounged out of a friend's basement, though I still washed my cloth diapers at the Laundromat. My parents sent me the towels and linens that we'd received as wedding presents, and my mom made me some curtains, a little bunting and a quilt for John Michael's room. I was by myself, but I had my baby, and I was back at school. It was enough.

## II

Most things I did as a mother that first spring and summer back at Dartmouth were based on things I'd read in novels. I'd read all of the *Anne of Green Gables* books, and Anne Blythe has six children. I'd read *Little Women*, and Beth takes care of the neighbor's baby, and *Little Men* in which Jo has her own children. I'd read Sylvia Plath's poems about her babies, "Love set you ticking like a fat, gold watch," Anne Lamott's *Operating Instructions*, and lots and lots of books by Noel Streatfield and Elizabeth Goudge in which British nannies held forth sensibly about the importance of exercise and a regular sleep schedule. I also went by instinct. I didn't like the smell of baby food, so I didn't use it. I steamed vegetables and mashed them smooth with a fork and a bit of formula, and my baby loved them. I knew that my tired, stressed body liked soft light and soft sheets, so I made sure my baby had them too. Every afternoon we took a nap at 1:30. Most nights we were both asleep by 9. Most of the time, we were alone.

Meanwhile, on campus, it was spring term and then summer term, 1991. I took French, Seventeenth Century Poetry and Prose, History 2, Earth Science 2, Shakespeare 1, and Modern British Fiction. I don't exaggerate when I say that the British Fiction course saved my soul. I had a spectacular professor, Brenda Silver, who gave me my first taste of Forster, Lawrence, Woolf, Conrad, and in particular, Jean Rhys's *Quartet*. Absolutely everything resonated. Loss of self and culture, sexual alienation, the complex tapestry of motherhood, personal and political anarchy – it all made sense in a way that was not at all academic. Outside I was still an embarrassed upper-middle-class girl with an improbable baby, but on the inside I realized I was as isolated by culture and gender as these writers' protagonists.

It's almost too self-consciously literary to note that a female dean took me to lunch and told me I'd never make it through the year without a full-time nanny. I tried not to think about my baby in class because I didn't want my breast milk to come down. My GPA those two terms was a 3.7.

Three other students brought children to Dartmouth when I was there. One was a tall, long-haired, Native American beauty whose child was rumored to have been fathered by a native African during an environmental study abroad program. Her name was Rachel, and she was already a senior when her baby was born. She took a term off, maybe, and then graduated a few months after her classmates. The second woman, a married student, had planned her children. She and her husband put each other through Dartmouth, trading off terms and slowly accumulating credits. I met them just once at a dinner organized by a dean. They both had dreadlocks and seemed awfully well suited to their Vermont lifestyle. The third, a girl named Jen, was the same age and year as I, and she, too, had chosen to marry the baby's father when confronted with a surprise pregnancy. She didn't return to campus as a student after her baby was born, although she came up to visit every few months until our class graduated.

Of course, I admired Rachel even though I knew I was more like Jen. I didn't have the cultural cachet to pull off a personal feminist revolution like Rachel's. She was proud, empowered, and her baby was a stunning biracial symbol of her social independence. I remember her telling me about her job offer at Episcopal. She hadn't told them about her child when she interviewed; she was pretty clearly looking forward to the shockwaves she was going to create when she reported for dormitory duty as a single mother. I was fascinated by her confidence and her conviction.

But I was a Christian, white, middle-class girl. So began the long, agonizing tension between my well-honed instincts for responsibility and my ill-fitting role as an untraditional parent – a reluctant foil to conventional family life. During my senior year at Dartmouth I spent holidays as an officer's wife at Fort Drum, New York. It was during the conflict in Somalia, and I was expected, as part of my husband's job description, to play a role in the "family support activities" while the soldiers were deployed.

While school was in session, John Michael and I lived with four of my best friends in a little house with three bedrooms just off campus. On Saturday mornings, John Michael would rap on my roommates' doors at 7 a.m., hoping for a playmate. We converted the dining room into a computer lab, and there I worked on my senior honors thesis, sometimes with a cranky two-year-old toddler on my lap. The essay, a long treatise on the medieval feminine ideal as it appeared in the works of Geoffrey Chaucer, is a wonder to me even now. Just shy of 100 pages, it is a complex, far-reaching, hilariously meta-critical opus that actually attempted to deconstruct the Virgin/Whore dialectic as it appears in "The Wife of Bath's Tale," "The Prioress's Tale," and the polemics of the early Church Fathers. It was exactly what one would expect from a Christian girl who had got hold of a little Derrida.

I still went to church every Sunday, and there the good, conventional Vermont housewives would invite my little boy and me to play dates, and to Sunday night dinner with their in-laws. When I was invited to sit on a prestigious feminist panel during my senior spring, again, John Michael was with me. I spoke passionately about what it had meant for me to keep and raise my baby in an environment unfriendly to mothers, and tried to elucidate issues I thought were going unnoted inside the politics of reproductive choice. I would have been more comfortable sitting in the audience, having my consciousness raised, and looking forward to an intelligent legal or academic career.

I graduated in June of 1993 – with honors, and in pearls. John Michael wore a little handmade suit and rode proudly on his father's shoulders. Our friends' mortar boards were emblazoned with the names he'd given them: 'Ty,' 'G'bar,' 'Sindee.' My whole family traveled to attend the ceremonies: aunts, uncles, cousins, and my sweet, smiley grandmother. At the party following graduation, the father of one of my friends, an investment banker who lived in New York City, interrupted the festivities to single me out from the other graduates for a toast. They all thought I had achieved something.

I didn't think so. The investment banker's daughter was on her way to a prestigious film internship in Manhattan. I was headed back to life as an officer's wife on a military base in upstate New York. All the feminist rhetoric in the world couldn't change my feeling that I had let myself down.

### III

In the spring of 1995, I had my second baby. Her name was Veronica. When she was about two months old, she and I and John Michael moved to Simsbury, Connecticut, to live and work at the Ethel Walker School. John was now a captain, having departed for a year-long unaccompanied military assignment in Korea. The children and I lived in three dorm rooms, joined together by a bathroom and a tiny galley kitchen. All the windows faced glorious east; it will not surprise anyone who has spent time with very young children to hear that it was a year of many exquisite sunrises.

Maybe it was because we were living in the fertile Farmington Valley, or maybe it was because I was again breastfeeding and single-parenting and thus tired and hungry almost all of the time, but my memories of that year are almost entirely of food and the seasons that influence food. For the first time in my life, I lived in a climate in which peaches and pears ripen on trees instead of in crates, in which a killing frost is not a certainty after the first of September. It was the year I discovered fresh basil and sun-dried tomatoes and the good nutty taste of mint and feta and couscous combined, the year I learned to bake bread, the year I first made jam. At night I'd nurse Veronica while John Michael made a meal of plums and rich, velvety yogurt that a tiny dairy was willing to deliver right to the steps of our dorm.

It was my first experience with the idea of a dining hall, and I loved that, too. I loved the feeling of plenitude, of course, and also that of community, the way friendships developed from sharing the same table night after night. Walker's is an all-girls' school with a staff comprised largely of women. There were babies and parents everywhere – people breastfeeding in the dining hall, dads handing infants off to moms between classes, my friend's two-year-old son hanging off the fire escape waving to the girls as they walked back to their dorms. During fire drills the girls in my dorm would show up at my door to carry one or both of the children. I loved the way that they jockeyed for their turn to hold Veronica.

I began, that year, to read Wendell Berry, Kentucky's beloved farmer/poet. I read him hungrily – his poems, "Farming: A Handbook," "Sabbaths," "The Wheel," his novels, *A Place on Earth, The Memory of Old Jack*, his essays, "What are People For?" I was ravenous for the metaphors of farming that suddenly made sense to me in a life that was filled to overflowing with stewardship and harvest. I loved the images of tilling and planting, tending and harvest, killing and decay, his seasonal metaphors, his laboring metaphors. "Harvest will fill the barn," he writes, "the hand must ache, the face must sweat." John Michael was already four years old; I was starting to know what Berry meant. And because Berry wrote about them in his essays, I read Harlan Hubbard, Edward Abbey, Norm McClean, John Steinbeck and Wallace Stegner – the epic American writers, lovers of land and place, describers of the cycle of death and rebirth.

It's very sweet – when I think about it – that I found a way, at last, to be at peace with my place within the deep, primal sweep of motherhood from reading the writings of several very serious white men.

We did a lot of walking that first year at Walker's. I'd put Veronica in her backpack and hold John Michael tightly by the hand. We roamed the horse paths behind the school's barns, and sometimes we'd drive down to walk in the farmlands west and south of Simsbury. In the autumn we'd bring home a bag of apples. In the winter we'd wear hats that I'd knitted during the three-hour faculty meetings held on Tuesday nights. By spring Veronica could demolish a peach while riding in the pack. I can still feel her sticky little hands in my hair.

## IV

When I took a job at Phillips Exeter Academy in the fall of 2002, I knew immediately that I was all but back at Dartmouth. The Georgian architecture, the oak furniture and polished seminar tables in Phillips Hall, the preppy, outdoorsy look of the students, were all familiar. And once again, there were rumblings about a war in the Middle East. John, now a major, was again discussing deployment scenarios with me. I was uneasy about the familiar turn of events and worried about starting a new job under the same kind of stress.

I knew, as well, that we were very likely going to end our marriage – our long friendship and mutual respect having endured better than our desire to continue our intimate relationship. Once again, it looked very likely that I was going to be on the wrong side of convention. I was heartbroken about this possibility.

Sure enough, John was deployed in dark January, and we soon knew it wouldn't be a short-lived conflict. For the first few weeks the children, now eight and twelve, and I walked around in terror, even though I did my best to block out the media barrage that surrounded the outbreak of the war. But there was the good hard work of juggling children's needs and meeting the demands of my teaching to do, and the familiar disciplines started to work their old magic. Each week I wrote our schedules on a piece of paper and posted it on the kitchen counter so that we would know what we would be doing – soccer games, basketball practice, dorm duty, class, meals, laundry, Ultimate Frisbee – and once in a while we took a long walk around the grounds, though this time one of the kids would wear the backpack.

For the first month or two we could talk to John on the phone. Later, when he was in Tikrit and contact was much more sporadic, the days were longer and at least we had the consolations of spring.

One of the things I did during the winter and spring terms of that year was develop a penchant for telling "bad mother stories" to my advisees. I told them about how, when we were living abroad, I sometimes didn't feel like taking the kids to school so I created a thing called "home school." On one home-school day the three of us ended up at the mall watching *Billy Elliot*. Lots of times we just went to the beach. I told them about how I hosted Veronica's birthday party and did not give out favors. I told my students about how I swore sometimes in front of my kids, and let them watch way too much *SpongeBob* and also *Futurama*, and about how we watched the WB show, *Gilmore Girls*, with a commitment that bordered on addiction. (My girl students were pretty enthusiastic about this last bit – by the end of the year we had between five or six converts watching with us every week.). I even admitted to them that I was often so late to pick up my daughter at the Main Street School that the principal told another mother that I was establishing a pattern.

My favorite bad mom story is one of several about how bad I am at helping my son get to school on time. It was the last big snowstorm of winter, in 2003. My son, who still dreads waking up for his 7 a.m. school bus, had rolled into my bed, fully dressed, backpack on, in all ways ready for school except that he was not at all awake.

"Just five minutes, Mom," he said. I was barely awake: I had dorm duty the night before. And it felt great to put my arm around my boy, who was too sleepy to shove it away as he does now, because he's twelve. So fine, five minutes.

About fifteen minutes later my own alarm went off, but one of us hit the snooze and we slept right through the bus. By the time we pried our eyes open, I knew I was going to have to drive him. We ate cookies for breakfast on the way out the door. My daughter joined us in our breakfast of cookies and was pretty stoked about it, and about the fact that I was going to have to drive my son to school. As soon as I was out the door, she would put on the TV – something she is never ever allowed to do in the mornings. "I'll stay here and wait for you, Mom. I don't mind," she said helpfully.

Outside it was still snowing, and the houses were panting puffs of breath out of their chimneys, and it was absolutely gorgeous. The only traffic was school buses and snowplows – their orange and yellow lights cutting through the fog of early morning at regular intervals. We were skittering through the slick streets in a half-defrosted car, giggling a little about how lazy and irresponsible we were, co-conspiring. I was doing this on purpose. It was good "bonding," I reasoned. Quality time. I decided to take a shortcut through the back roads to the middle school. It would be faster and prettier, I told my son, who snorted at the word "prettier."

I really thought I was making a shortcut – even though the ride had already taken ten minutes longer than it should have.

And then we started giggling about whose fault it was that he would be late. Neither of us was paying attention, and before we realized it, signs appeared announcing that we were at Hampton Beach. We were completely lost. We giggled even harder when we thought how we were going to explain how we got lost on the way to a school that is a mile and a half from our house – a school that my son had attended for seven months. Even so, we didn't consult a map or ask for directions. We just turned around and went back along the long, circuitous route by which we came, looking out the window into the slowly opening day.

I was driving slowly on purpose. John Michael was on the cell phone to Veronica laughing and telling her how we still really didn't know where we were, and how we were all going to get into big trouble. I smiled as he spoke because we were together and I was not alone, and I was not ashamed. I knew at last that I was not at all a bad mom because we were driving around in the sweet, lush spring snow just as lost as we could be ... and just as happy.

# MOTHERWRITER

## *Barbara G.S. Hagerty*

I took to the art of writing instinctively. The art of mothering has come harder to me. And for many years, these two activities – one introverted, the other extroverted; one a solo act, the other, at minimum, a duet – seemed to arise from different psychic impulses and belonged to parallel universes. I naturally separated them. The surprise has been in how they have come together.

First, I became a writer. I was a nerdy, dreamy kid, a walking train wreck of ophthalmologic anomalies and introverted tendencies that can create a bookworm. I had strabismus, astigmatism, myopia – conditions and words I didn't understand, but which rolled around provocatively in the fertile landscape of my imagination. My lazy eye gave me an inward expression and I lived out its silent directive, learning to look inward at meaning, symbol, metaphor, and word, long before I knew the vocabulary of introspection. I was clumsy at sports, bored silly with volleyball, tetherball, basketball – not a team player. Early on I realized that I was an outsider and that language was my natural habitat.

When I was six, a small but transformative thing happened to me. A local journalist read a short paragraph I'd written for the school literary magazine, liked it, and arranged to have it reprinted in the local newspaper. On the day that my words appeared in print, I became hooked. No doubt my addiction arose partly from the intoxication of seeing my first byline, but I believe it is more complex than that. It was seeing proof that the idea – the necessity, even – of formulating and articulating one's viewpoint and projecting it to a larger world was possible. On that day, I was like Ben Franklin standing in the rain and lightning with his kite and his key.

What's so mesmerizing about spending the whole day in a room alone, with just the company of words? It's the limitless, unpredictable meander of the imagination, the infinity of possibilities, the surprises delivered from various regions of the brain: memory, hunch, and inspiration. Take a fork in the path, wander into a cul-de-sac, or fall down the rabbit hole. Set off in one direction, take a detour, and end up someplace strange and new. Ever inward. Our frantic culture meanwhile exhorts us to get up, out. Carpe diem! But I have always secretly belonged to the Emily Dickinson School of Thought. For the writer's life IS the life of the omnivore. As someone – Augusten Burroughs perhaps – said recently, "Leaving your room is highly overrated."

I was much entrenched in my writing lifestyle – a confirmed soloist who worked at home, with a hard-working, hardly-ever-home man to have dinner and sleep with every night – when the first of our four, much-wanted, much-adored children came along. Yet, if I came to writing like a merganser to a pond, mothering was more difficult, a fish on a bicycle kind of thing. I did not enjoy pregnancy and found my one experience of natural childbirth horrific.

Such was my introduction to motherhood, an enterprise that for me swung between holy and holy hell.

The learning curve toward competent motherhood was steep. Overnight, I became a mother, and overnight, reverie, free-spiritedness, independence, and peace and quiet disappeared. Eventually my self-absorption dwindled and I discovered in myself the capacity to enjoy raising children whose ages could be expressed in double digits. But all that happened slowly and over time. As a thirty-year-old new mother, I worried constantly that the artist in me would disappear under a pile of dirty bibs and crib sheets. Suddenly I was getting up several times in the middle of the night, boiling pacifiers, cranking up the Swing-o-Matic, and retrieving Cheerios from under the sofa. Instead of reading *The Golden Bough*, I was reading *Goodnight, Moon*.

I was unprepared for the wise tyranny of biology when just five days postpartum, I made a lunch date with a colleague. I had barely touched my quiche Lorraine when my milk let down, my concentration faltered, and my body commanded: Go home!

Yet, somehow I persevered through my long, on-the-job training, learning to juggle a child (later, children) and freelance assignments, cutting back on work, taking more on, as the demands of life ebbed and flowed. Eventually I settled into a terrific gig, as a monthly columnist for SKIRT! Magazine for its first five years. My support system was exceptional: regular sitters, a helpful, hands-on husband, a mother and a sister who lived five blocks and eight blocks away, respectively. Nonetheless, well into my older children's teen years, I still thought of myself as having two personae: one, that slightly bohemian person, the artist, the loner who stood slightly outside the culture; the other, the mother whose job was just the opposite: to carry the culture forward, both through the birth process and later via actual trips in her minivan.

From time to time I fantasized what my life would be like if I did not have the responsibilities and encumbrances of a family. What if I did not have to cook meals for six on a daily basis, settle sibling disputes, sit through long games in the gymnasium, call out vocabulary on flash cards, or find someone else's missing shoe or lost jacket at 6:30 a.m.? What if each day were a luxurious tabula rasa on which to paint words, eat a carton of yogurt for dinner, sleep whenever, read for hours at a stretch, talk to fellow artists, daydream, or entice the muse? What would it be like to be able to call one's time wholly one's own?

When the kids were in high school, I had my chance to find out. Rounding up my best writing samples, I applied for a competitive fellowship to attend an artists' colony for two blissful weeks. My application was bolstered by the recommendation of a novelist friend, much established, who had insight both into my work and my hectic life as a mother of four. I never read his letter of recommendation, but he once told me the gist of it: "if any writer could benefit from two weeks at a writers' colony, it's this woman." (Translation: please take this beleaguered mother in and give her asylum!)

The utopia I arrived at some months later – suitcase and laptop in hand, expectant as any first grader on the first day of school – consisted of a complex of buildings clustered on an expanse of pastoral land. Beyond its boundaries, sweeping out to the far horizon in every direction, were hundreds of acres of rolling blue-green farmland. About twenty writers, visual artists, and composers were in residence at any given time. I was shown – as each Fellow was – to a private, Spartan bedroom with cinderblock walls, a single bed, and reading lamp. A few hundred feet away, a second room awaited me: a private studio for uninterrupted work. Nirvana! There were no schedules to follow or chores to do and I can recall no rules other than the sacred dictum never to interrupt another Fellow at work. One could simply disappear into one's art, if so desired, but most of the Fellows did come together for communal breakfast and dinner in the dining room. After dinner, we'd write down what kind of sandwich we wanted for tomorrow's lunch and turn in our orders to the kitchen. The sandwich would appear in a metal lunchbox, as if by magic, outside one's studio door at the noon hour the next day.

Full of talent, ego, ambition and invention, the hilltop colony vibrated, thrummed, practically levitated with around-the-clock creativity. It has sheltered and nurtured over 3,000 artists in its time; among them are winners of the National Book Award, the Pulitzer Prize, and the MacArthur genius award. The writer in the studio next to mine was putting the finishing touches on a novel that would become a play on Broadway (*Wicked*). There was a cross-dresser among us, and one artist who painted in his own blood, puncturing his veins daily and collecting fluid in a vial. I wondered if my scarlet letter, "M" for Mother, showed and felt sure I was the only one in that heady Camelot who could be counted on for cupcakes and carpools at home.

During those two weeks, I concentrated by day on a collection of poetry I had assembled over the years; evenings, I spent in the colony's darkroom, working on a series of black-and-white photographs that were published in book form three years later. But mostly, I worked on myself. Or the place worked on me, in ways I could not have anticipated.

It's funny when you at last get what you think you want. My two weeks in that greener grass were cool, productive, and revelatory. I reworked poems, printed photographs, took walks, napped, talked, thought, and read, read, read. I played poker a couple of nights with the other artists, attended occasional readings, visited open studios, and made a few friends.

But I also crept down to the basement several times and used the pay phone to call home and reconnect. Once again, the emotionally wise tyranny of biology had kicked in. To my surprise, I found that I missed – ached for – the messy complications of life, the interruptions, and the human encumbrances. In a word, I missed my family. I had underestimated the ballast that they were in my life. I had not understood how they enhanced, rather than subtracted from my work. I had not realized that through being part of a family, I had fundamentally changed. The girl with the lazy eye, the competent parent, the bookworm, the artist, the community member, the carpool driver – I knew I was, without contradiction, all these people. Identity, as I finally came to understand at the writer's colony, is not a case of either/or, but rather of both/and. On that hilltop, I realized I had grown up, and my personae had fused. I had, at last, become motherwriter.

*Originally printed in Literary Mama, February 2009.*

# THE WORM BIN

*Nina Misuraca Ignaczak*

The worms are dead. They were supposed to have been my recycling machines, turning carrot peelings and lettuce heads to garden fertilizer, providing an educational science experiment for my kids, teaching them about waste and efficiency and the circle of life. More than that, they were supposed to have been a tiny step toward making a commitment to creating a more sustainable life for my family. Now they have become the very compost they were supposed to create. And it is all my fault.

There was a time, in the unspoiled ideology of my early twenties, when my values aligned perfectly. I was an environmentalist and a feminist. I planned to cultivate an egalitarian marriage, pursue a career, have kids, and foster a healthy connection to the earth in my family and community.

I became a feminist first. In the suburb where I grew up, most families looked like mine: an overworked, stressed-out father, a stay-at-home mother who functioned variously as grocery-getter, laundress and chauffeur, and two-point-five kids per household. My mother bought me a hope chest for my sixteenth birthday, where I would store old copies of *Sassy* and *Ms.* magazines. My father was a respected attorney, and despite having no mafia ties, identified with Tony Soprano to an alarming degree. His favorite Tony Soprano quote: "It's 2000 and whatever outside, but in here it's 1950."

My girlfriends and I, sunning ourselves in our bikinis around the municipal swimming pool, would roll our eyes as we listened to the young moms prattling on about their husbands' latest business trips or promotions as they fed crackers and grapes to their whining kids. We made a pact to shoot each other if we ever ended up like that.

Later I became an environmentalist. I studied natural resource management in college, which led to my job as an environmental planner for a government agency. I married my college sweetheart, and we spent our twenties pursuing our careers and taking exotic vacations. When I turned thirty, I gave birth to my first child, a healthy and "spirited" boy who didn't sleep through the night for a full year. He made me crazy, and I loved him more than I have ever loved anything.

My life plan was on track – marriage, kids, career. I never expected that my return to work post-baby would be filled with such tremendous anxiety and sadness. I left the daycare center on most days with tears blurring my vision. I grew weary of lugging the sleekly designed yet cumbersome pumping apparatus downstairs to the women's shower room at my office, explaining to co-workers why I needed to leave my desk at inopportune moments. At home, we were drowning in laundry and starving for a decent meal. My husband was traveling to Europe and Asia every other month for extended periods of time. I was alone and overwhelmed.

When my second child arrived a year and a half later, I hit the wall. I was having a hard time sleeping, eating, even getting out of bed in the morning. My stomach was perpetually in knots. I started taking an antidepressant and tearfully tendered my resignation.

Fortunately my supervisor was able to shift me to part-time, giving me two full days each week to spend with my kids and enough compensation to make it worthwhile.

Life has settled to this side of tolerable. On the flip side, I have not exercised in months, I catch every bug that goes around in daycare, the laundry in our house is piled to the ceiling, and I am still carrying around the weight from my second pregnancy.

My twin values of feminism and environmentalism, which once seemed to fit together like a hand and glove, now seems more like a foot and hat. This cognitive dissonance manifests in a particularly stark manner about once every other week, usually on a Thursday. After spending my day writing grant proposals for energy efficiency projects, working with a local watershed council on stormwater management, or mapping local food resources in the community, I pick my kids up from daycare and strap them into the minivan. They are famished and crabby and I am exhausted. Of course, I have forgotten to plan dinner. My husband is working late or is out of town. The Golden Arches loom in not one but three separate locations on our path toward home.

Soon the chant begins. "Chicken Nuggets! Chicken Nuggets!"

It is here, waiting in the drive-through line at McDonalds, about to hand my kids sacks of chemically-laden frankenfood complete with advertising gadgets masquerading as plastic toys, that I have the most serious internal debates about the course my life is taking.

Perhaps that is why I installed the worm bin in our house, as an attempt to reclaim the "eco-feminist" buried deep within the shell of a tired, working mom. It was a gift from a local woman who runs a small "intentional community," a sort of hippie commune in which people live and learn about green building and other sustainability skills. When I arrived to pick the bin up, she apologized for the fruit flies, which swarmed from the bin in great clouds. The fruit flies followed us to our kitchen, where they innocuously floated around as the bin filled with banana peels and lettuce cores. When the flies finally multiplied past our tolerance level, we relegated the worms to the backyard. It was early April in Michigan, and on the second night, the temperature dipped below freezing. The tropical worms froze to death in their bin.

The eco-feminists of our day make valid points. They claim that public policy can achieve only limited impact; for real and lasting change, we need billions of people willing to alter the way they personally live, work, and consume. And yes, this will need to start in the home. Domestic skills such as childcare, gardening, cooking, and making things yourself are proposed as salve for an ailing world.

Yet I find myself unable to wholeheartedly embrace the exhortation to "renounce, reclaim and rebuild" when I think about the implications, not least of which is losing the opportunity to contribute professionally to something I care deeply about.

Together, my husband and I have managed, through trial and error, compromise and collaboration, to devise ways of sharing the burden of running a household while maintaining two jobs outside the home. There is much room for improvement.

The worms do not always survive. But so far, the kids have.

# A FOOT IN TWO WORLDS

*Lindsey Mead*

When I was twenty-six, and one year out of Harvard Business School, I attended a social event held by the school's "network of alumnae." It was a small group in someone's home, and a classmate and I were, by ten years, the youngest women there. At one point, the women began talking about their struggles to balance their professional and home lives. I was married but childless, and the challenges they described seemed so distant as to be indistinct on the horizon.

Despite my inability to directly relate, the tone of the discussion bothered me. The women were negative, full of complaints about the ways in which they had to trade off one thing for another on a daily basis. One made a comment I've never forgotten, the gist of which was that everybody thinks you make some large, symbolic choice – once, showily and finally – between your children and your job. She said that it was, instead, a choice she made every single day in a thousand small ways.

For some reason, I spoke up. At a break in the conversation, I tentatively cleared my throat and asked, "Well, I don't want to overstep here, and obviously I don't have kids so I don't know, but ... ," I hesitated, "isn't this kind of a great problem to have? Isn't this a privilege, ultimately, to be choosing between a job you love and children you love?" I was roundly dismissed for not knowing how hard it was and for opening my mouth without any actual understanding of their plight.

And, of course, we were both right. I know that now, after seven

139

and a half years of trying to find the right balance between my two children and my professional life. I didn't know then what I was talking about and probably ought not to have said what I did. Still, I believe to this day that having both a career and a family that you adore is one of the world's great problems.

I haven't ever had that job I love, though I have tried for many years to find it. To keep open the option for the day I do, I've been unwilling to give up on my professional life, though it has comprised jobs that never felt particularly challenging or rewarding. Neither have I been willing to give up the flexibility to spend time with my children, during the week, during the day. So I have spent these years trying to be a mother with a career who is also home with her children. I acknowledge that it is a great good fortune to have this choice at all, and that this is a dilemma of privilege.

After deciding in January to leave my part-time job at a private-equity firm where I managed recruiting, I began interviewing with executive search firms. The process triggered a landslide of self-doubt. I realized anew how little I feel I have accomplished in the decade since I graduated from business school. I have chosen a path of having a foot in both worlds ("career" and "home," both in quotation marks because I think these definitions are simplistic), and as a result I have a home in neither.

What does it mean to have a foot in both worlds? I think it can be wonderful or it can be torment, depending on the person and the situation. I've always straddled the gulf of the mommy wars, always worked part time, always spent part of my week in an office building and part in the sandbox. I have insisted on keeping a "foot in the door" professionally because I was sure I'd want to "ramp back up" someday. These phrases, so familiar in business school, seem foreign on my tongue now, like a language I used to speak but have lost. The thing that haunts me is this: In being unwilling to give up either world, did I end up doing a poor job in both?

I decided when my daughter was born to scale back my professional aspirations and involvement in order to have more flexibility to be home. And still I ache about having missed the babyhoods of my daughter and son. I wonder if I would feel better about my children's infancies had I chosen to be home full time – if I would feel I had inhabited more of those swollen, bittersweet moments that dot my days as a mother. It's easy to blame that on the fact that I was at work some of the time, but when I'm honest I don't think that is the reason at all. I think it's about my wiring, my frantic restlessness, the way I struggle to be fully engaged in one thing at a time.

And yet I also feel frustrated by what feels like wasted years, spent only partially engaged in jobs that, in retrospect, did not mean very much to me. To keep the flexibility I prize so highly, I have chosen roles that are often peripheral, not core to a company's function, and I have been an individual contributor rather than a member of a team. This has eroded both my sense of making a real contribution and of feeling part of a cohesive group. What was the point of having missed hours with my babies for something that feels so insubstantial and inconsequential now? Of course, the dirty truth is that I didn't really *want* to be there every single second.

People comment over and over again on how well I've figured out how to have a flexible, part-time career. And when people say that, I always smile and nod and express my satisfaction with my situation. But I haven't figured anything out, and those comments always make ambivalence and regret roll into my heart like thunder. They remind me of all of the anxieties and misgivings I have about the trade-offs and choices I have made.

My friend Aidan has written about how she frets that she has wasted her education. I relate to this. I worry that I am letting down my parents, who made an enormous financial and emotional investment in my education. I worry that I am failing the teachers who took a particular interest in me, made me believe I was not stupid, helped open my mind. I don't feel that I am letting down those people because of my specific choices, but because of who I am: because I am not more curious, ambitious, intelligent. I am certain that the fears of disappointing these role models are a big part of what spurred me to keep working all of these years. Yet can they really be proud of such incremental efforts, such minimal achievements in the professional world?

Some days I feel that I'm the epitome of that saying, "a mile wide and an inch deep" – that I've skimmed the surface of many worlds but not had the courage to pick one and immerse myself in it. On other days I think that I am simply more kaleidoscope than laser. Those days, when I am feeling kinder toward myself, I think a life splintered into myriad pieces fits me because of my manifold interests. I think that I could never commit to one place, because I never found one singular place that felt like home.

*Originally Published online in PAW (Princeton Alumni Weekly), September 22, 2010.*

# MOTHERHOOD AND METAMORPHOSIS

*Kim Todd*

When I discovered I was pregnant, I was knee-deep in research for a book on an adventure-loving woman who, 300 years ago, at the age of fifty-two, sailed to South America from Amsterdam to study insects. My desk lay buried under notes on Maria Sibylla Merian and her pioneering investigations of metamorphosis, the change of caterpillar to butterfly. Stacks of books detailed how she and her peers, at the dawn of science, explored questions of development and transformation. How does a creature gain new parts, either a human embryo growing lungs or a caterpillar sprouting wings? They wrangled with the enigma of self divided. Larva and moth. Mother and child: Were they one, or two?

Suddenly, the mysteries probed in these seventeenth-century treatises were unfolding under my skin. Within weeks, my hair developed a luster beyond the magic of the most expensive conditioners. Insomnia, a clean, hard light bulb of wakefulness, switched on reliably at 3 a.m. A three-mile run had been part of my routine for years, but now I was limping back, gasping, after a few blocks. A trip to the ob/gyn not long after revealed that I was breathing not just for two, but for three. Twins.

And those were just the obvious changes. At the start, the embryo is only the smallest packet of cells hitchhiking in the uterus. In the intervening months, though, the placenta pumps out its own hormones, ordering the mother's body not to cast off the uterine lining. Only a thin cell barrier separates mother's blood from fetus's, and oxygen and nutrients slide across it. Near the end, the belly dimples and its occupant kicks at stimulus the mother doesn't even feel. How to parse out these threads of interdependency?

Lying awake in the dark, feeling for the twins' heartbeats, I was afraid not so much about altered blood vessels and shortness of breath, but a loss of psychological oxygen. In this sea of new swells and fluids, was there still room for some flinty core of self? I had always worried that a career as a writer, with its low pay and non-existent health insurance plan, would be expendable once I got married and had kids, an artsy affectation easy to shuck off in the face of family life. As I fretted over this in high school, wondering if I shouldn't take physics instead of more English, my sister, ever the pragmatist, said "Kim, right now, nobody wants to marry you."

But, eventually, someone did. The concerns flared up again as I tried to lull myself back to sleep night after night, imagining both forward in time to when the children would emerge, and backward to see Merian and her world. Her history was obscure, except for flashes provided by a letter, a sketch, a recorded conversation. The uterus, like history, was unknown except for the skeleton view provided by the ultrasound and the ripples as an arm or a leg skimmed under the surface. I found myself glad that the fetuses were not alone in all that darkness.

During the day, I lugged my belly to the library. Waddling through the stacks, I saw all the more clearly the obstacles Merian faced – married with two children, a woman loaded with domestic tasks, financial responsibilities, and a desire to pursue this strange fascination with insects. At age thirteen, she painted a watercolor of a silkworm: its eggs, caterpillar, pupa, cocoon, and moth, and it launched her on a journey that would last for more than fifty years. Others looked at the insects at each separate stage, dissecting them under a microscope, but she wanted to know how they moved from shape to shape. Over the course of her career, she wrote and illustrated five books – one about flowers, three about European insects, and one about insects in Surinam. She painted watercolors and taught classes and captured and sold reptile specimens. My

144

original research questions had to do with Merian's notions of metamorphosis, her role in her scientific community. Now, as I sat at the table, breathing hard after the short flight of stairs, I was more curious about how she'd found time and energy to paint.

The economy of seventeenth-century Germany relied on women. Household industries depended on them to sell vegetables, keep accounts, tend livestock, and run a weaver's loom. A printer's daughter, like Merian, would have engraved book plates and mixed watercolors. Three hundred years ago, as today, women sought to balance childcare with earning money, though Merian was perhaps unique in the way she let her own interests dictate her labor.

But she made it work. When her daughters, Dorothea and Johanna, were young, she experimented in the kitchen, counting maggots that hatched on larks waiting to be cooked for dinner. A wasp's nest "large as a man's head" found in a Nuremberg attic was ripe for investigation. When she moved back to Frankfurt to care for her recently widowed mother, a sloe branch swathed in a velvety communal caterpillar nest proved too tempting. She broke it off and set it up in a room in her house so she could watch it change hour by hour. Even her father's gravesite offered insects for her collection. She plumbed the habitats of daily life.

And when the time was ripe and her daughters grown, she moved beyond these domestic investigations, to go where no one had gone before. The South American rain forest threw tight webs of vines and dense thickets in her path, and she hacked her way through them.

The twins were born in February, the umbilical cord cut. At times, looking at my newborn son, with his round green eyes and my daughter with her little Irish mouth, both traits from my husband, I couldn't imagine we shared any genes at all, much less that my breathing had once fed their blood. As they turned in sleep, responding to dreams without language, they seemed inhabitants of a different world.

My body shrunk to roughly its original contours. But with the flesh no longer divided, the mind split, busying itself with a new set of baby anxieties even as the book deadline grew closer. My husband, Jay, and I adjusted to life in the infantocracy, setting the alarm for nighttime feedings, drawing up and scrapping schedules, making endless rules to limit the chaos. The most important rule was this: If both children are crying, no adults can cry. Hard to follow, but vital.

Finally I had to get back to it, and when the twins were four months old, we all went to Europe to retrace Merian's steps – her childhood in Frankfurt, her young married life in Nuremburg, her middle-age career move to the Netherlands.

Sleep-deprived already, none of us were braced for the jetlag that hit in our first few days in Amsterdam. My mother's cousin lent us her attic room, complete with two bassinettes. As rain rattled down on the skylight, the twins squirmed and babbled as if it were noon. At some point, Jay and I gave up urging them to sleep and just let them play on the bed, trying to hold onto enough consciousness to keep them from tumbling to the floor. The next night was no easier and Jay, cradling Ben, trying to soothe him, said, "Here I am, holding my son, with my wife, in Amsterdam. I can see myself looking back on this moment, thinking I wouldn't trade it for anything. But right now, it stinks." Ben arched and whined in rebellion, and the hours slid on toward morning.

Afternoons, groggily, we toured as a family, and I picked up my sole word of Dutch: *tweeling* or "twin." Passersby repeated it as we monopolized the sidewalk with the double stroller. When we all visited the Rijksmuseum, it became apparent that my son found the sound of the language hilarious. As the guard cooed at him, his ringing laugh drowned out the tour guide's interpretation of the Vermeers. My daughter, who liked bare feet no matter what the weather, left a trail of kicked-off socks throughout the city.

Mornings, I set off on my own. At the university's biology archives, I pored over original Merian watercolors. In one, a cut hawthorn branch stretched across the parchment. Amid the creamy white blossoms and blood red berries, insects crowded the page. The browntail, the goldtail, the tussock moth, spread their wings over the twig crawling with caterpillars. Eggs, pupae, and cocoons nestled in every available cranny. It was messy and animated, alive as a heartbeat. This close, sketch marks showed underneath the paint, all the necessary adjustments and revisions.

The collection also had a rare copy of her last insect book, a record of her research in the northern Netherlands and Amsterdam, a project she labored over until right before she died. This final volume of worms on hazelnuts, gray moths and their eggs, notes on a nest of ants, showed the markings of two different, though related, authors. As Merian grew sick, her younger daughter took over, engraving the plates using her mother's watercolors as models, arranging details of publication. Merian's notes of a green and white caterpillar eating rose leaves, turning into a pupa, and then hatching into a fluttering brown and white moth, were brought to life by Dorothea's artistry, her insects larger than Merian's, her pressure on the engraving tool firmer, the emphasis on grays rather than black and white. The two lines, that of the mother and the daughter, blended on the page. Two hands merged back into one.

Back on the balcony of the Amsterdam apartment, I lifted my daughter to touch the geranium in the window box, petals all the more red for being slicked with rain. Across the courtyard, a woman bent to her tiny garden, every inch of soil in this land-poor country bursting with flowers. My girl was so slight, her bones felt hollow like a bird's. A butterfly landed on a leaf, and she reached for it with fingers barely able to do her bidding. I blocked her hand to save the insect, and she squawked in protest. So light, so full of will.

We were both tender in our new forms. Pregnancy and motherhood bring weakness, stillness, a disorienting loss of control. To shift so dramatically, in the middle of life, seems like a liability. My daughter wriggled; the butterfly lingered; and Merian came to mind. Her biography is a model of how to work within constraints, to grasp a vision tightly, refusing to let go in the face of jarring events. But her watercolors chart more than this: not just the strain of weathering all these changes, but the joy. More than a map for survival, they are a tribute to transformation.

She captured all that the caterpillar gains by its different guises: its mouth is shaped to eat leaves when leaves are plentiful; its mouth disappears when it tucks itself away in a chrysalis; its mouth turns to a long proboscis to suck nectar when it lives the flitting life of a butterfly. The ability to alter, to move from singular to plural and back, is the insect's greatest strength. It has the flexibility to creep and hide at certain times; to become liquid and immobile; then eventually, like the one that launched itself off the balcony into a gray, Netherlands sky, to soar off on gaudy wings.

*Originally published online at LiteraryMama.com, August 2007.*

# MORE THAN "JUST" A MOM

*Jennifer Ulveling*

"You're lucky, you don't have to worry about any this. You're married. You're thin. You're completely put together. Your life is probably perfect!" The twenty-seven-year-old woman I see twice a week for psychotherapy dissolves into tears. I see her pain, the complete, aching loneliness that overwhelms her, and her desire to find "the one" – a perfect mate so that she can end her time in purgatory and finally begin living her life.

My client is sobbing in front of me, and I am lost in my own thoughts, wondering what she would think if she knew the feats of dexterity it takes for me to get my kids to daycare in time to meet with her twice a week at 9 a.m. Today, I managed to arrive with just one sticky jam hand print on my blouse, which I have carefully hidden under a scarf. I have become an innovative dresser, between frequent stains and infrequent dry cleaning runs. I also wonder if she had any idea how many more hours I clock in deep conversation with her than I do with my own husband each week. My marriage is stretched so thin, it feels as though even one thoughtless look might break it.

When I started seeing this client a year and a half ago, my youngest son was five-months old. I expressed breast milk for him in the minutes I had between appointments. I would close the office door, hang an "in session" sign on the handle, and pray that no client would walk in to find me half naked, attached to a breast pump.

During that same period, my three-year-old son was having difficulty sleeping on his own. He would creep into my closet and take dresses and sweaters to sleep with – new ones each night that would end up in an ever growing heap under his covers – a pile of transitional objects, in psychological terms.

He would never take the cotton "mom" t-shirts. It was as if he understood that a small part of me existed for myself, not solely to care for him, and he wanted to be with that part. Between finding clothes that were not wrinkled and drooled on by my older son and something that allowed for easy breast pump access for the baby, dressing each morning in my sleep-deprived state became some sort of gateway test to determine if I was competent to leave my role as a mother and engage in the professional world.

I am now interning as a psychotherapist three days a week – unpaid, tired, and stretched physically, emotionally and financially. I pay more for childcare than I make in a counseling session. My schedule is clustered into micro-intervals. I spend time training, seeing clients, marketing my practice and commuting between various venues. I do my best to nurture my maternal side by baking cupcakes for birthday parties and making homemade Valentine's cards with my children. As my psychology training has taught me, I do my best to be emotionally present for my boys, not just feed and bathe them.

My only time to myself is at midnight, when I sneak downstairs to watch *This Old House* on television. I love *This Old House* because I know that it will not be emotionally draining. They always get it right the first time. They are competent, even masterful, as they build and fix houses. I love watching the insulating foam as it expands to fill up the open crevices. There is something deeply satisfying about watching it grow, pushing out the air until the excess goo oozes back out through the holes in the wall.

Last week I picked up the boys from our nanny's house after an emotionally draining day of seeing clients. When I arrived, they cried for ten minutes straight in a desperate duet of pure exhaustion. My husband was out of town, and our schedule had been thrown off kilter. Unfortunately for all of us, we had to stop at the grocery store to pick up milk and something for dinner. As I pulled the boys out of the car, I was hovering slightly above barely functioning.

I knew there was little chance that we would make it in and out of the store smoothly. Two cranky boys, a ragged mom, and the bright lights of the supermarket combined to guarantee nothing short of disaster. As expected, we had meltdowns in every aisle – battles over potato chips, who got to put what in the cart, and what kind of candy they wanted but weren't going to get. We were one person away from checking out when my four-and-a-half-year-old looked at the overweight woman in front of us and asked loudly, "Mommy, why are her legs so big?"

Maybe if I had gotten my PhD, I would have had the perfect answer to my son's question. But armed only with a master's, I did not. I mumbled something about it being the same reason as why some people have blue eyes and some have brown eyes, why some people have blue skin … um pink skin … and some have brown skin – people are just born different. This answer seemed to satisfy him. He turned his attention back to repeatedly asking why, in our family, we are never allowed to buy candy in the checkout aisle.

I went back to study psychology, in part to gain insight into my innermost self. Through my studies and my own personal therapy, I have regained access to a more youthful, creative part of me. I have begun to write poetry again, to take joy in dancing crazy dances with my kids while we do the dishes, to find that I care deeply about my place in the world. This feels like the real deal to me; I want to tell everyone, to give everyone this gift.

What I did not realize when I left a lucrative legal career to go into psychology was how it would provide deep, painful glimpses into parts of myself and my marriage that I did not want to see. Nor did I realize how much my husband would be along for the ride. Now, a few years into my new career, we have learned more than we would have cared to about ourselves and each other. Although we have been fortunate to manage financially on one salary, we are both stymied by my "neither here nor there" status. I am working, paying for day care and school, yet not earning anything. I often feel selfish, with two young children who need clothes and books and lessons and college educations. I know it is something that I need to do, but I also know that my husband's support for my choice is waning.

Giving up my current career would most likely restore some balance in our lives and our relationship. But when I became pregnant and had children, something in me seemed to stand up and demand attention. It insisted that I not be subsumed into the deep feminine well of motherhood. This part of me – the independent career woman who fought to be viewed as an equal, the Princetonian who loved learning for learning's sake – demanded not to be lost when I moved into parenthood. I know that I need more in my life than just being a mother, especially a mother to young children.

The strain on our marriage is palpable. My career "redo" causes my husband to confront his own ambivalence about his job. He questions why we are investing time and money in a career that will never pay what I earned as a lawyer. He has always earned more than I have, and there was never a question as to the necessity of his paycheck. With all of our bright ideals and shiny views of gender equality, our marriage from this vantage point feels eerily like something out of a past era.

In a manner similar to the insulating foam on *This Old House*, my new passions – being a mother and a therapist – are expanding to fill every crevice of my time. They have swept the excess away, and my husband and I struggle to make sure that we make enough time to focus on our relationship and each other.

I am also reminded of that foam each morning when my two sons climb into bed with us. We start each day as a family, squeezed into a bed not big enough to contain the body parts, big and small, that snuggle and wrestle and kiss and hug. We are one big pile, and everything that isn't loved or loving is pushed out. These moments remind me that, though I struggle constantly to find balance, I have created a life where the moments of happiness more than compensate for the difficult therapy sessions and grocery store meltdowns. If I can manage to hold my marriage together through all of this, I will consider myself one of the most fortunate women I know. But keeping it all together is delicate balancing act. I wrestle with the reality that I may not succeed, and how little this may all mean if that proves to be the case.

# WHEN I SNEEZE, I PEE A LITTLE

*Windi Padia*

When I was seventeen, I remember asking my idealistic Baby Boomer father if I would have to choose between a career and a family when I grew up. "No," he said, "those days are gone. You can be whatever you want to be and have a family, too." He made it sound so simple, as if all the obstacles holding women back had been wiped out by his generation, leaving only a wide open path for me. He left out the small detail that becoming a working mother would require more energy than any one person can be expected to possess. But how could he know? He was never a working mother. I've learned to forgive him.

The two most important factors in my decision to marry my husband were the calluses on his hands and the fact that he talks very little, unlike the Ivy League men I went to college with. He's a game warden – a wildlife cop with a gun, a badge and a biology degree – like I used to be. For me, being a game warden was not a job. It was a lifestyle fueled by adrenaline surges. I imagined the stories I would tell my grandchildren as they gathered around my rocking chair. I would start with the time the poacher hid the mule deer cape from me; how I had a hunch something was wrong because of the nervous way he picked at his clothes when I inspected his muzzleloader; and how that hunch led to an interrogation, two search warrants, and his confession of poaching not one, but three deer. I'd tell them the one about the bear stuck in a tree near a school, how I ignored the camera crews while I loaded drug darts with shaking hands, then climbed onto the roof next to the tree and tranquilized the bear as he tried to jump onto the roof with me. Those lucky kids. Their grandmother was such a fine example of a woman.

I'd been a game warden for three years when the undeniable urge to start a family hit me. When I became pregnant, I expected that I would be able to compartmentalize my life. I pictured two of me: Windi Warden and Windi Wifie. Windi Warden was fearless and persistent, rather like pregnant Detective Marge Gunderson from Fargo, waddling across a frozen lake, gun aimed at the bad guy. Windi Wifie was a homemaker who painted and organized the nursery, read the correct books and did smart exercise routines. She found time to spend with her husband.

Instead, Windi Warden was simultaneously nauseous and ravenous. She was irked that her breasts were too big for her bullet-proof vest, even with stretchy fasteners, and annoyed that her duty belt wouldn't fit after just five months. Fatigue would hit at the ridiculous hour of four-thirty in the afternoon. She'd drive around in her pick-up truck, barely awake, and find herself on the wrong side of the road. Windi Warden was so tired she could not physically work more than fifty hour weeks. And Windi Wifie was cranky if she couldn't go to bed by eight o'clock. Finding a place to pee consumed her dreams. She cried during the last scene of *The Goonies*, a movie she'd seen dry-eyed about a hundred times, when Data's Dad called Data "his best invention."

I wondered how I could possibly mix demanding work hours with a new baby. I considered finding an easier job. When I told my boss I was pregnant, I knew our conversation would be bigger than just him and me. It would be a statement to the world that somehow I was less of a game warden. I planned for the conversation to be a casual "heads up, boss, I'm pregnant" sort of thing, but by the end of our talk, I had made the decision to go on light duty – no law enforcement – and had asked my boss if he knew of other jobs for me. I became obsessed with money worries – a job requiring fewer hours would surely pay less. I made a list of the pros and cons of continuing to work after the baby was born. On the pro side was "work life continues" and "combined income," and on the con side was "baby will be emotionally scarred for life." One night my husband put his hand on my belly and said, "Our investment is in here, not in the amount of money we make."

My boss made some phone calls and found me an office manager position at the regional office. I would lose my status as a game warden and spend my days helping customers and answering phones, but would earn the same amount of money working forty hours a week instead of seventy. An old game warden who had taken me on horse pack trips found out about my job change. He cleared his throat several times, betraying his emotion, when he told me he thought I could have a child and still be a good game warden. On the books, my job move was officially called a voluntary demotion. I had the sense, and so did my coworkers, that I was taking a step down. I would no longer be working long hours, a sure way to get promoted, so I lowered my career expectations.

There is a stigma on moms who put their babies into childcare, who do not feel the need to spend entire days gazing into their children's bright eyes. My parents were surprised at my decision to continue to work full time after the baby was born. I wondered why they sent me to Princeton in the first place. I wondered why they bought me the three hundred dollar breast pump. As much as the new mom books told me that giving birth and breastfeeding were the ultimate culmination of what it meant to be a woman, there was a part of me that wanted to succeed in a career, to have a life of my own. Even if we could have kept the same standard of living on one salary, I did not like the thought of being a full-time mom. There is a stigma, especially in Ivy League circles, on career women who give up their jobs for their families. When I told one of my college friends that I was pregnant, she was shocked and reminded me that being a mom would ruin my career. It amused me because I was so ready to be a mother, yet I was thinking exactly the same thing she was. When the baby was born, my husband took a month off of work and I took three months of maternity leave. I had this crazy notion that I had to be perfect at everything, and since I was a woman, breastfeeding would come as naturally to me as a summer breeze to a waterfall in the misty mountains of unicorn land. It took two sleepless weeks until I was comfortable with it. Immediately after that, our baby began crying for no reason. He would be fed and changed and warm and dry and would launch into heart-rending screams that made me want to throw him out of a second-story window.

Months of getting up often in the middle of the night to pee had prepared me for an erratic sleep schedule, and I had enough energy to feed the baby every two to three hours. My husband, on the other hand, felt like he was sitting around watching us, waiting for the little guy to get hungry. If a man can get the baby blues, I think my husband had them. I cracked a book about fatherhood and discovered that most men do not feel emotionally attached to their children until their kids are walking and talking. Furthermore, sometimes a couple can go through rough times because their only focus becomes their baby and they forget the work it takes to keep up a marriage. I was putting all my energy into our baby and shutting my husband out. I was not letting him be a father, but I expected him to be a cheerleader for me on the sidelines.

After my husband went back to work, he would come home in the evening from ten hour days, during peak crying hours, and take the baby so that I could have time for myself. I looked forward to going back to work and felt guilty for looking forward to it. I wondered if it was fair to my son that I was pining away for the relative quiet of an office.

When I dropped my baby off for his first day of daycare, he was hungry. He drooled on my black shirt while the teacher got his bottle ready for him. I gave him to her, and she sat down in the rocking chair, cradled him and put his bottle into his waiting mouth. He grabbed her fingers and closed his eyes. It broke my heart.

Despite having given up my game warden job, I kept my law enforcement commission. On my first day back on the gun range, I spent seven hours shooting my handgun, rifle, and shotgun. The inevitable rush of milk into my engorged breasts brought me back to the reality of my new life, and I searched for a place to pump. The only private spot I could find was a port-a-potty, and I just couldn't bring myself to untangle the tubes and wires of my breast pump in there. I considered sitting in my car with a jacket over my shirt and pumping while the other game wardens walked back and forth, but decided I couldn't risk the embarrassment if a well-meaning coworker approached my car to chat. I went nine hours without pumping and developed mastitis. I missed work for two days because of the infection, which knocked my sick leave hours back to zero.

The whole theory that changing jobs would be bad for my career was wrong. Although I have traded my hiking boots for high heels, I am able to work fewer hours and still make more money than I did before. I work from home two days a week. I've been promoted, twice. I have nights and weekends off and spend them with my son, often just the two of us, while my husband works. My supervisor – a working mom herself – leaves little calendar pages on my desk that say, "How can we teach our children the value of solitude if we do not take time for ourselves?" She has introduced the strange concept that working long hours proves nothing, and is not the only path to success.

I read somewhere, maybe on a calendar page, that the key to being a working mom is to partition the brain. When I am at work, I should think only of work. When I am at home, I should be fully present to enjoy every minute of my child's discoveries about the great wide world. When we have a babysitter and I am on vacation with my husband, I should think only of our romance. This idea appeals to me – it is wonderful. Windi Worker, Windi Wonder-Mom and Windi Wifie all refuse to let their worlds overlap, and yet coexist in harmony. I have no idea how to make this a reality. I do know there needs to be a fourth woman: Windi. Just Windi, independent from everyone else.

My husband struggles with this multiple identity question too. He is a working father. I do not mean that he is a father and he works; I mean that he is a man who juggles work and family just as much as I do, if not more. He works more hours, but the hours are flexible, so he is frequently the parent at doctor appointments. He takes our son to daycare in the mornings and picks him up when I have a meeting that runs late. He works extra hours on the weekend to make up for the time he spends with our son during the week. He's going through this right along with me, minus the major body overhaul. I'm the one who has to pee every time she sneezes.

Momhood is full of conflicting emotions. I experience anger and frustration at being pulled in a million directions, plus this bewildering gratitude that, at the end of each workday, I get to hug my son goodnight and put him safe and warm in his crib, and then fall asleep while my husband holds on to me like I am his anchor, and not the other way around.

# PLATO AND MODERN MOTHERHOOD

*Regan Penaluna*

"I'd rather be making cupcakes!" said my sister.
She said it so many times, in fact, that our mother had it printed on a T-shirt for her birthday. Cupcakes to my sister meant spending time at home with her baby. Before she gave birth, she had set out to become a scientist. Yet now that her baby was here, she wasn't so gung-ho. In truth, my sister did not want to stay at home baking cupcakes all day, any more than she wanted to be working all day as a scientist. But splitting her time between the two was not that simple.

My parents raised us with the belief that we could "be anything we wanted if we only put our mind to it," and now my sister found herself of two minds: she wanted to be a mother raising her baby, but she also wanted to be a successful scientist. Like many modern mothers – myself included – she could not do one without feeling as though she was significantly shortchanging the other.

Plato would not be surprised. Even though he was writing over two thousand years ago in ancient Greece, entirely unaware of the modern woman's condition, he said a few things about motherhood that were interestingly spot on. Or, at least his character Socrates did in Plato's most famous dialog, *The Republic*.

In this work, Socrates proposes to build a city from scratch in his mind. Many wild things come of this, such as a eugenics program to annihilate all persons over age ten (as, at this point, they are "corrupted by tradition") and a "noble lie" told to citizens to get them to accept this program. Socrates' willingness to vastly reconsider many aspects of society also leads him to a somewhat forward-looking take on women. Challenging Greek tradition, Plato has Socrates pitch the idea that women have the same "souls" as men, by which he means that they have the same mental capacities. As such, women can reason and so are capable of vocations typically reserved for men, like politics and philosophy.

To persuade his friends that a woman can do a man's job, Plato argues that it's absurd to allow one's physical appearance to determine his ability to do a job. Take hair length, for example. He says that, "if bald men are shoemakers, we won't let the longhaired ones be shoemakers, or if the longhaired ones are, then the others can't be." Socrates wants us to consider that other physical traits, such as one's sex, should not necessarily decide one's professional destiny. Just because women are physically different from men doesn't mean they should have different jobs.

But what does this all mean for motherhood? Socrates wants women to be mothers (smart women have smart babies, he assumes, which is good for society), but he also wants them to keep their jobs. His solution? "[T]he children … will be in common, and neither will a parent know his own offspring, nor a child his parent." He proposes breaking the mother-child bond "so she won't recognize her own." As early as 380 BC, Plato was presenting us with the idea that women could be mothers *and* professionals. In Plato's world, however, these women would not feel torn between these two worlds, like some of us moderns. By teaching women to see their own children as common to all, Socrates conditions the mother out of them. Literally.

Getting rid of the mother's soul, as Socrates does, is not a solution for me or my sister or any modern woman for that matter. And Plato didn't really seem to think it was a solution for ancient women either. There are suggestions throughout his text that he made the creation of the city so absurdly impossible that he didn't really wish for it to exist. What we *can* say is that the difficulty Plato saw facing women – that they are smart like men but also by nature drawn to care deeply for their children – is probably why every morning, as the legend goes, he thanked the gods for having made him "a philosopher, an Athenian," and foremost, "a man."

Before my son was born, I looked forward to the connection that I would feel for him. Everyone told me how the parent-child bond was so unique. Yet I also harbored a deep-seated fear that this love would diminish my professional drive. Somewhere lurked the belief that the more time I spent with him, the weaker my ambition would become. After I became pregnant my mother liked to tease me about my earlier proclamations: "I will never marry!" and "I will never have kids!" Perhaps these were attempts to "get the motherliness out of my soul," as Socrates might say.

I did get married, and now I have a child. Like my sister, I also want to enjoy staying at home and making cupcakes, yet that desire is easily overcome by my drive to do other things. I get an undeniable joy from both my maternal and professional sides, That still doesn't resolve the wrenching I feel in both directions. Living with that is better than the alternative Socrates offers.

*Originally published online at The Philosophers' Magazine, November 19, 2010.*

# Part Five

# Give Me a Break!

ദ്ദ0ദ0

*Break clear away, once in a while, and climb a mountain or spend a week in the woods. Wash your spirit clean.*

– John Muir

# DR. MOM

*Tara Bishop*

Exhausted after a long day spent chasing my two-year-old son around the park and nursing my three-month-old baby every two hours, I collapsed on my bed. Just as I was drifting off, I heard the sound of dishes being shifted on the table. My eyes shot open and my head jerked up. "Honey, I'll do it," I called out to my husband, home from his thirteen-hour work day.

"Don't worry," he said. "I'll just stick 'em in the dishwasher and crawl into bed with you."

I should have felt grateful, but what I felt was guilt bordering on panic: I should be doing those dishes. That sinking feeling has become a common one in my new life as a doctor turned stay-at-home mother on what the *New York Times* and several recent books dismissively refer to as the "mommy track."

Several months ago, I was working full-time – actually, more than full-time. I had an eighteen-month-old son and was slowly rising in the ranks of doctor-hood. I worked sixty-hour weeks, often evenings and weekends. I wasn't happy. In fact, I was miserable. I felt extremely guilty for not being home more with my son (even though he seemed happy spending his days swinging in the park with a very loving nanny). I was stressed – constantly struggling to keep my home life afloat. But I was on a secure path to a high-flying career and had figured out ways to keep my life organized – order groceries on Tuesday to be delivered on Friday morning, work on my research project at night after everyone else had gone to sleep.

Nine months into my first year of fellowship, I unexpectedly got pregnant again. Instead of being overjoyed, I felt overwhelmed. With the pregnancy test in hand, I turned to my husband, tears blurring my vision, and asked how I could keep doing what I was doing with another baby at home.

He wrapped his arms around me, and said, "You don't have to."

On that cloudy April evening, I decided to quit my job. There wasn't even a debate over who should stay home. My husband made more money than me in his finance job, loved going to work and never felt guilty leaving our son.

I wasn't completely comfortable quitting my job, so I told people that I was "taking a break." In fact, I was embarrassed to be wasting an undergraduate degree in chemical engineering from M.I.T. and a medical degree from Cornell. Before my son was born, I read the "Opt-Out Revolution" in the *New York Times* and saw a *Sixty Minutes* segment about highly educated and successful women who gave up their work to be home with their kids. At the time, I vowed never to sacrifice my career.

Five years later, I found myself doing exactly that. The first few weeks at home were a series of adjustments. I went to the playground and tried to become friends with other stay-at-home moms. I beamed as my son played his mini guitar better than all the other kids in his music class. I loved that I once again had time to read novels.

But I was also very, very bored. I would spend hours each morning trying to get my son to sit on the potty. I would answer his endless "why?" questions. By the end of the day, I was dying to talk to anyone who could complete a sentence.

To fight the boredom, I began to apply my Type-A personality to motherhood. If I was going to be at home full time, I figured, I would be the best damn stay-at-home-mom ever. I started watching the *Barefoot Contessa* daily on the Food Network and bought Martha Stewart's home-keeping bible. I made daily trips to buy antibiotic-free, locally raised, free-range chicken. I created a spreadsheet to compare all the Upper East Side nursery schools.

And while I'm not quite as compulsive these days, I continue to feel, every day, the weight of the brainpower I'm not using.

Whenever I talk to former colleagues, I wonder if I can still read an EKG or diagnose pneumonia. I look forward to trips to the pediatrician because it gives me a chance to discuss the latest research on autism and vaccinations.

While some may argue that the "Mommy Wars" are still being fought in our society today, I don't see any overt battle between stay-at-home moms and working moms. All I see is a war each of us fights within herself. Before I had kids, I was great at my job. After having kids, I felt mediocre at everything: doctor, mother and wife. I wasn't willing to be middle-of-the-road, so I made choices.

"Choice" is the fetish word of our generation. We are the generation that took pride in the fact that we could break the glass ceiling or devote our lives to our children; society would accept anything. But it won't. It's very difficult to work overnights when you're breastfeeding. There's always pressure to work more. So we have to give up something. And if you're a woman, that usually means neglecting your kids or your career and feeling guilty either way.

I have no doubt that I made the right decision to leave my job. But I miss being a doctor. My new plan is to go back to work when my sons are in preschool, but not on the ambitious track I was on before. With luck, I can find a more reasonably paced job. I expect that will mean retiring the fancy cookbooks, missing some of my son's music classes and not always washing the dishes. This level of compromise I can handle. And that's what I think about in those moments when I am convinced I can't face another sandbox, another diaper: one day I'll be part of the working world and still able tuck the kids in at night.

*Originally published online at Babble.com, 2007.*

# STARTING OVER

*Amy Hudock*

Today I turned forty years old.
    I hold in my hands the gift I received on my tenth birthday, an orange and gold plastic earring case. I remember back to that day – how I got up, fed the horses, and went for a long ride through the pine forests near our North Carolina home. As the trail broke into a sunny meadow, I eased Rainyday into a canter and dropped the reins, holding my arms out to better feel the wind we were moving through. I felt like I was flying.

On the day I turned twenty, I went out for beer with some friends at Henderson Street, a Chapel Hill bar that was popular with the Kappa Sigs. I ate popcorn from the ancient machine at the corner of the bar and drank the cheap beer. When I got back to my dorm that night, I couldn't sleep, so I got up and went for a walk. I knew girls shouldn't be out walking the campus alone at night, but I didn't care. It was silent, except for the echo of my footsteps in the empty colonnades that framed the stately buildings around me. I stopped to watch the windows of Wilson library mist over – low interior lights falling in patterns on the bricks at my feet. I imagined the books in the reading room, sitting on their wooden shelves that ran up to the doomed ceiling. I felt I could do anything, go anywhere. I was powerful and strong.

I turned thirty years old in an art-deco house built from the plans of the *Good Housekeeping* Stan-Steel home, one of the "homes of the future" displayed at the 1933 World's Fair. The house was owned by two of my friends, and we gathered there with a group for wine, artichoke dip, and pesto. I was a new assistant professor in English, and along with other new professors, we drank toasts to our careers, to possibility. One of my favorite pictures was taken at this time, one I keep framed on my desk. I am sitting in front of the black marble fireplace, wearing a cowboy hat and jeans. A glass of red wine sits next to me. I am not smiling, but the look on my face is bold, confident, and hopeful. As head of a committee to start a Women's Studies program, I thought I could remake the world.

Now, on my fortieth birthday, I can't sleep, so I write with a pen I received from a fellow mother-writer friend. It has weight to it. Its color is the kind of green that makes me want to taste it. I feel that I can write more, better, because of the pen. My friend helps me mark the change of life by honoring what is important to me now, as I turn forty.

I haven't ridden in years. I can't take late night walks because my daughter (and social services) might object to her being ousted in the middle of the night. And the friends who were hired with me in 1995 are going up for full professor this year. I've come full circle, returning to the same place I had been nearly twelve years ago when I had just completed my PhD. Now I am starting over again in the same department as a visiting assistant professor.

Back in 2001 I contacted my department head with the news that I was pregnant. When I requested maternity leave, he replied, "You've already had one year's leave to teach at Berkeley."

"But this is maternity leave," I said.

I emailed him a copy of the Family Medical Leave Act to convince him the law was on my side. After reviewing the document, he told me that, according to the law, they were only required to give me a few weeks leave. He told me the date he wanted me back, which would mean driving across country in mid-winter with a newborn infant, no husband, and no help. Regardless, this is what was required if I wanted to keep my job. I had to make a "choice," he said.

I thought of it as a "choice" back then, too. The "Mommy Wars" had framed the debate in this narrow, either/or way. I could choose "career," or I could choose "family." Not both. As a woman who had started and run a Women's Studies program, as an ardent feminist, the choice should have been clear. I learned from women of my mother's generation the major lesson – don't ever give up your career.

When I was young, my divorced mother cared for us during the day and waited tables at the Holiday Inn at night when we were asleep. I remember going into the kitchen cupboard one afternoon to get something to eat and finding a can of creamed corn and some bread. That was it. Later that week, I found my mom crying at the kitchen table as she sat over a small pile of money that she tried to spread among too many envelopes. Eventually, we left North Carolina and moved into my Grandmother's house in New Jersey so we could survive financially. My mother felt incredible pressure to marry again so that she would have help. I never wanted to be in the same position.

In choosing to put my career first, I had given up so much, left so many people I loved behind, and committed myself to a solitary existence, except for my dogs and cats and the occasional boyfriend or roommate who moved their things in and then out. Loneliness was as much a part of me as the dull ache from my once-broken wrist. Quiet. Gently painful. But always there.

It's unnatural for humans to be alone. When I met my future husband, a man who was like me – enlightened, liberal, and a professor – I felt he was a "good risk." He was a single father of a fifteen-year-old daughter, having lost his first wife to cancer. A man who knew how to take care of himself and nurture someone else. I thought feminism had largely eradicated the inequities in marriage – especially a marriage to another PhD. I felt safe.

So in the spring of 2001, pregnant and thousands of miles away from home, I decided to stand up against the conventions that demanded that a successful woman "have it all" – career, family, and an independent income – and resigned from my full-time, tenure-track position. Feminism was about choice, after all, and I was choosing to stay home to raise my newborn and my stepdaughter. I believed, somehow, that the lesson I had learned from my mother was no longer applicable. I knew I was strong. I knew I would find another job later, once the baby was older. I knew I wouldn't face any discrimination because of my choice. I believed I could have it all.

Things didn't turn out quite so rosy. Although my husband had seemed like a "new man" at first, once the baby came, it was all over. I never expected to hear him – or anyone in my life, for that matter – say, "Where is my damn clean underwear?"

It became like 1950 in our household. When I challenged him on his archaic definitions of gender roles – "If you need it right now, wash your own damn underwear" – he laughed at my feminist pretentions and told me that he made the money; my role was to clean the house and do the laundry and care for the child.

I didn't walk out. I knew I should have. But I had no job. And I was across the continent from my family and friends. I tried to make it work. I read *Buddha Mom* and explored the Zen of housekeeping. I attacked my internalized negative stereotypes cluttered around the image of women's traditional work. I struggled to raise the value of doing laundry in my own eyes, but found it hard when I knew only my hands were doing it.

I resented him for leaving his cereal bowl on the table after breakfast, for creating messes that he then blamed me for not cleaning up, for making cleaning up after him a command rather than a request.

His outrageous, irrational, angry outbursts over housekeeping came more frequently and with more ferocity. When he began throwing things and threatening divorce, I put my foot down.

We entered counseling. Yet counseling only served to clarify the gendered conflict over work inside and outside the home. He was angry at me for leaving him as the sole support of the family, for putting pressure on him to stay in a salaried position rather than going out on his own as an individual consultant. He told our therapist I compared badly with his first wife, who was a successful trial attorney and still kept a perfect house, kept his clothes clean and put away, and kept the child. To him, I was a failure because I needed his help, though he seemed to forget his first wife had a full-time, live-in housekeeper and childcare provider. I sat quietly through most of these sessions, stunned into stillness. I was unable to articulate my sense of betrayal.

In our second-to-last session with our therapist, my husband called me "stupid" for giving up my job. Finally I exploded. I saw it all then in ugly, painful clarity. I was no longer an equal, and thus not as interesting or as desirable as I once had been. He didn't want me anymore. He had married a successful, independent woman, and he no longer saw me as that. I saw myself through his eyes, and that person bore no resemblance to who I was once. I had become a housewife. And he hated me for it.

A few weeks later, I packed my bags and left with my daughter for South Carolina, where I had taken a job as a visiting assistant professor. My husband helped us settle in then returned to California, where he started his own business and filed for divorce. Suddenly, I was the sole income provider. By leaving my tenure-track position years earlier to raise my family, I had forever interrupted the course of my career.

I should be at a certain rank and salary with a nice retirement fund by now. But I am not, and I don't. I am back on the job market looking for another tenure-track job, but I am not making enough money to support my family.

I have become what I never wanted to be – the mother hunched over the kitchen table with too few dollars for too many gaping envelopes. I feel the panic of knowing my income is not enough. I take my daughter to her preschool each day, thinking, "Please, let her like it. Let her be okay," because I know she has to be. She has to stay there. I have to go to work. I have no other option.

Once I thought that U.S. feminism emphasized individual economic independence too much as a reflection of our money-focused community; I was wrong. We cannot emphasize it enough. No one is really safe in a country where over fifty percent of marriages end in divorce. When I consider my life now, the concept of "choice" has a whole new meaning. I should have listened to my mother. I should not have imagined I was immune to the forces that shaped her generation. I should have known that opting out is not a real option; it is financial suicide. And I should have known better than to put the noose around my own neck and call it a choice.

# EVEN A SUPERHERO NEEDS A BREAK

*Ashley Stone*

At some point in every *Batman* flick, our sexy and plastic-clad hero returns home. He sulks, shuffles and drags his dilapidated bat mobile into the Bat Cave. He's down, but not out. He needs to recoup and rejuvenate, ready to take on the next bizarre and twisted villain to come his way. It's usually in that pivotal part of the movie that the moral becomes clear, and with that clarity comes victory. It's something like being a mom – not just a mom, but Super Mom.

You remember her, right? She can leap over a mountain of laundry in one single bound. She has organic cereal in the cupboard and well-kempt and oh-so-polite children lined up and ready for school each morning. Unfortunately, she hasn't had time to face the mound of laundry in three days because she's been too busy running from school to home, to baseball practice, to swim team, to ballet, to choir, to the post office, and to the supermarket. The minivan is losing its bat mobile disguise due to lack of washing, and the super kids don't look so clean anymore, either.

At the end of the day, when all kids have been collected and accounted for, Super Mom heads home. She hauls the younger ones upstairs to the tub. She considers using a washcloth, a singsong voice and a game to wash her children. Instead she grabs the removable shower head and hoses them off, a little squirt of soap here and there ... done! She quickly grabs the PJs and, after several attempts at putting the right one on each kid, she gives up and tells them to figure it out themselves.

She then speed-reads a story, kisses them goodnight and turns out the lights. As she walks down the hall, her hand pressed to her temple, it all begins to fall off. First the cape flutters dramatically to the ground, then the seam that's been awfully stretched blows in the rear end of her tights. Her meticulously coiffed hair tumbles to her shoulders, revealing a stripe of gray roots that have yet to be dyed and a flurry of split ends that she keeps to give her hair volume. Our heroine is tired, lost, and broken. She loves her life and her family but she's desperate. She NEEDS a break!

I'll let you in on a little secret: the kids are only clean because those Mr. Clean Magic erasers really do work on anything. And the organic cereal boxes? Those have been filled with Fruit Loops. She's just trying to keep up appearances. And truth be told, she struggles some days to actually remember her children's names. It's become easier to refer to them by their numbers, like Dr. Seuss's Thing One and Thing Two, since those numbers coincide with the information on the calendar that helps keep her organized. She's actually thinking of getting t-shirts made with their numbers on them for Christmas.

It seems sometimes that we as moms feel we need to do and be everything for everyone, to keep all the balls in the air, and do it with grace. And while we're told again and again that it's okay to not "do it all," there's a bigger issue to face. We need a break. Not the kind of break that means leaving your husband and children behind forever, not the kind of break that means seriously rethinking your life path, but the kind of break that leaves you refreshed.

The hard part about needing that break is that as Super Moms (don't kid yourself; if you have children you manage to care for, provide for, and love, who are happy, you are a Super Mom), we feel it's a chip in our armor to ask for help.

In fact, the asking for, needing or even dreaming of such a break is our Kryptonite. It falls under the same category as not "doing it all." We feel inferior; we feel like frauds, we feel as though we are letting someone down. At least that's how I feel. I have a hard-working husband who is tired after a long day, and the last thing I want to do is ask him to help me when he gets home. Even though

I've had a tough day, and didn't sleep much the night before because the baby thought it would be sweet to practice being a teenager and decided to party at 3 a.m., I still feel a pang of guilt at the idea of asking for some time alone.

What if someone thinks I'm not doing this right? What if I let someone down? What if my husband is too tired, falls asleep, my three-year-old gets into the makeup and manages to turn her one-year-old sister into a better version of Dennis Rodman? What if? What if? WHAT IF?!

You know what? What if you took an hour? What if that hour consisted of tea and a book, alone? What if that hour was a walk in the fresh air at a speed faster than a snail crawls? What if you went to shop for pants and didn't need the handicap change room to accommodate your stroller, your children, their crap and yourself? What if you put yourself on the charger to reboot? The answer? You'd be refreshed. You'd have a chance to digest your days, your moments, your frustrations, and your fears. You might hash it out with a friend, or think quietly to yourself. You might smile a little more, because you've had time to think things through. You might look 5 years younger because the roots are now gone, thanks to a fabulous dye job and scalp massage. You might just find that the world keeps spinning even when you stop.

I think that as busy, working moms (and I mean working in the "living life with kids" sense, not the business office way; either way, if you have children, you're working: All – The – Time), we get so wound up in our schedules and our lives that our days become something of a cyclone, constantly spinning around us. And after a while that spinning starts to feel as though it's the earth's momentum, and we are the only ones holding all together.

But the real truth is, life goes on even if the laundry doesn't get done. Life goes on if instead of doing dishes right after supper you play with your kids and then go take a bath, with the bathroom door shut! Your husband – you know that guy who managed to have his life together enough when you met him that you decided to give him a chance and marry him – can actually hold it all together for an hour or two. Even if he doesn't quite do it the way you would, and Kid #1

– whose name is actually Thomas – may wind up with grease behind his right ear, but it's all okay, because they're safe and that detachable shower head is good for more than one thing.

You'll come home, come out of the bathroom, and return to the situation better than you were before. You might smile instead of scowl when your daughter breaks out into "The Song that never ends," because you haven't heard it in the last hour. Your attitude has taken the adjustment you're trying to get your teenager's attitude to do and you actually like being a mom, a Super Mom.

But what will take the cake – be the super-power recharge that you need – is what happens in those first few moments after you've arrived. Kids #1, 2 and 3 will come peeling around the corner, and amid shouts of "Mommy! Mommy! You're home!" and "I missed you, Mommy," and "How was your break, dear?" you'll feel it – that moment when the Kryptonite has been removed and Superman's wounds have healed. You'll feel loved like no other, needed like a cold drink on a hot day, and your littlest one will say, "I love you Mommy. I'm glad you're home!"

# A YEAR OFF

*Jill Gott-Gleason*

The other day, as we discussed my eagerness to go back to work after a year off, a friend teased me about "coming out of retirement." Taking time off to nurture my kids and my husband was important to me, but it was hardly what I hoped retirement would be like. Forget about tanned skin and Florida sunshine. Instead, I went from working 9 to 5 to working 24/7, 365 days a year. No paid vacations, no sick leave, and no sneaking out of the office for lunch with a friend.

Of course, there were some blissful mornings where I would find myself in the backyard, sipping coffee at 9 a.m. in my PJs, watching the kids jumping and playing and squealing. And I would think, "Wow, this is the life! How did I get so lucky?" And then, just for a second, I would replay the past two or three hours in my mind: My eldest child up at the crack of dawn with a wet bed ... Back to bed after changing PJs and sheets, only to be startled awake half an hour later with screams from the youngest child, weighted down with a big poopy diaper and showing no signs of going back to sleep ... Breakfast served at 6 a.m., complete with spilled milk and cereal, and arguments over whether to watch *Elmo* or *Caillou* ... Attempts to get myself dressed at 7 a.m., thwarted by tantrums from children wanting to go outside and play before the sun is fully up ... Another diaper change, another tantrum, and then, ahhhhh ... the coffee pot clicks off, and I pour my first cup, two hours into the morning.

It's more than fair to say that I had no idea what I was doing when I quit my job. I had no clue what my next steps would be, how we would pay the bills or survive the next year. I had changed careers four months earlier and wasn't far into my new job when I realized that I was thoroughly unhappy. So much, in fact, that I would cry while putting on makeup, dreading work like a child dreads a week at summer camp. I would feel like retching as I left for work each day. At the office, I would watch the clock moving ever so slowly and count the minutes as they passed. I knew I had to get out. But the money held me hostage.

One morning I did it. I quit. I can only imagine my husband's thoughts when I called him and told him the news. It was a release for both of us – a big exhale on a situation that had been about to explode – and yet at the same time it was horrific and scary. I emptied the desk drawer of personal items, a package of microwave popcorn and some lip gloss. I took the one picture I had of my kids, closed my laptop, and never stepped foot in that office again.

The most difficult part of quitting for me was that, despite hating this particular job, I actually enjoyed being a working mom. I never thought of myself as a stay-at-home mom, nor did I wish to become one. For me, the title Career Woman held more value than either Mother or Wife. Maybe it was my subconscious feminist tendencies. Equal rights. Equal pay. I can work. I can contribute to society. This was simply a detour on my path as a working mom, and I would be back on track soon enough.

Although I wasn't sure of my next career steps, I made sure not to burn any bridges with my children's daycare or stop bringing my clothes to the dry cleaner. I didn't want anyone to get too comfortable with this newly accessible mom, wife and friend. I was going back to work, after all.

The first month off was great. It was the honeymoon period. I was welcomed with open arms to a whole new group of women, the stay-at-home moms. We planned play dates and visited the mall for coffees while the children romped on the indoor play equipment. I was able to make dinner for the family each night and grocery shop during the day. I made the beds in the morning and tucked each child into bed at night. I could sneak in a nap here or there and even catch up on daytime television.

Then, about a month into it, I asked myself, "What the hell am I doing?" I started missing grownup lunches where peanut butter and jelly were not on the menu. I missed dressing up in more than sweatpants and having a reason to wear makeup. I craved voice mails and emails and deadlines and using my brain.

I tried to write, but I became lost in my overwhelming boredom. My sentences sounded something like this: "My mind is full of cobwebs, like the corners of my home." I would play with the kids for a while and look at the clock and realized that only three minutes and eleven seconds had gone by. I locked myself in the bathroom to escape the sheer boredom and simultaneous chaos that mothering two preschool-aged children can bring. I didn't know how to be cool, calm, and collected. I didn't know how to keep these kids or myself busy. I felt all mismatched inside. I loved my kids, but I missed the "up and at 'em" mentality of the working world. I found it hard to slow down my head and my heart to match the silly pace of toddlers. I realized that I couldn't function without running at 110 percent.

Friends and family would ask me how it was going now that I was staying home. On bad days I would lie. Play up the advantages and not tell the truth of how crazy I was feeling. On good days I could be honest and laugh lightheartedly about the bad.

When I became a mom, I never aspired to be one of "them" – a debit-card-carrying, minivan-driving mom. And now here I was. One of them. They looked at me sympathetically when I told them I used to work, their eyes saying, "God, aren't you glad you escaped from that?" And I looked at them sympathetically when they told me they never wanted to work again, my eyes saying, "Aren't you going crazy at home?"

The stay-at-home moms would chuckle nervously if I told them I was bored, as if it was daring to admit something so painfully true. They would ask questions like, "When you were working, who made your husband's lunch?" and "How do you ever finish all the laundry?"

I referred to my fellow stay-at-home moms, somewhat patronizingly, as the "stroller brigade." I was amazed at the way public spaces during the week were littered, literally, with hundreds of strollers and crying kids – shops, parks, museums. I never knew this world existed ... or at least I had never experienced it before. Women in sweats, pushing their precious cargo, in single, double, even triple strollers. Didn't they get the memo that kids can walk by the time they are seven?

I tried hard to understand these women. I learned that what made us different was what made us the same. They found answers to their lifelong questions in motherhood, and I, in a boardroom. And that was okay.

After I joined the "ranks" of stay-at-home moms, I came to better understand them. Like a frog in a pond with other frogs, we all knew it wasn't easy being green. We could let our kids scream without bothering innocent bystanders. We could say "no" to candy, toys and other unnecessary items in the checkout line and mean it. I came to respect them for who and what they were – sweatpants and all. And despite our many differences, I learned that in our hearts, we are very much the same. We work, we stay home, or we find something in between to keep us busy and happy. We crave love, sleep, chocolate, and a clean house. At the end of the day, if we can laugh and smile along with our children, we have done our jobs well.

Just the other day, I left the house in my sweatpants – the sweatpants I had actually worn to bed the night before – no shower, hair crazy and kids barely passable. I went to a store and then to a restaurant. I laughed and played with my kids. We were happy. All of us. I smiled to myself, realizing how far I had come.

# A DATE WITH MYSELF

*Sara Debbie Gutfreund*

I stand on the balcony and stare out at the mountains. It is so quiet here I can hear myself breathe. I can hear the birds softly chirping and the rustle of the flowers that sway gently in the late afternoon breeze. I feel my hand reaching for my cell phone.

I forgot to remind my husband about the baby's eardrops. I forgot to tell him that Shani doesn't like cream cheese in her sandwich anymore. And what if he doesn't remember that Ephraim won't go to sleep without his blanket? Will he remember to defrost the lasagna for dinner? Will Kayla remember to clean her newly pierced ears without me there to remind her?

But my cell phone is tucked into the closet, and I don't want my husband to feel like I don't think he is capable of taking over. He is probably fine. Besides, the sign in the spa said: No cell phones and no children under the age of sixteen.

It is too silent here. Almost eerie.

I decide to walk along the red cobblestone path that circles the hotel grounds. As I walk, I revel in the stunning sunset and the fresh air. But, after a couple of minutes, I begin to feel uncomfortable. Here I am, free to finally take care of only myself – no one whining, no one pulling on me, no meals to cook or laundry to throw in the washing machine, no lunches to make or noses to wipe ... just me. For the first time since my wedding, I am all alone, and I am shocked to realize that I don't know how to speak to myself anymore.

Could it be that, despite all my achievements as both a professional and a mother, I don't even really like myself? I try to shake that thought from my mind and enjoy the beauty all around me. After all, I reason, I am a very happy person. People turn to *me* for advice.

But as I allow the silence to penetrate my mind I allow myself to admit the unadmittable. I don't like myself. The frightening part – it shoots at me in the middle of this field of pastel flowers in the middle of nowhere – is that I have no idea why.

With all the noise and hectic pace of everyday life, it is always so easy for me to ignore myself. And for some reason my master's in psychology always keeps me confident. *Healthy, loving marriage* – check. *Happy, growing children* – check. *Warm, clean home* – check. *Nutritious meals and spiritual atmosphere* – check. *Happy mommy?* Well ... Mommy is content. For some reason happiness seems like too tall an order.

I want to run. I miss running. I miss speed. I miss exhilaration. I peer around me as if I am about to sneak a forbidden piece of chocolate. "No one is here," I whisper to myself, and I begin to run. Slowly at first but then faster, through the trees, past the tennis courts. I run faster until I cannot breathe, until I am one with the wind and the setting sun and the soft, green grass. I run until I can no longer see or think or feel, and then I stop.

I realize that for the first time in a long while I feel ... alive, and I ask God, "How can a person who wants to climb mountains stand in a kitchen and make scrambled eggs? How can a person who longs to run for miles and miles sit in the living room and help with homework, clean up spilled milk and change endless, dirty diapers? How can a person who graduated from an Ivy League university, who wanted to save the world, who spoke in front of hundreds of people, how can she spend most of the evening packing lunches, setting up outfits, reading bedtime stories, saying Shema, reading another story, getting another cup of water, and just one more story and ... now the baby is up. What do you do when you would rather go skydiving than wake up sleepy children, make breakfast, brush wayward hair and walk to the kindergarten on the corner?"

As I sit there on the edge of the field, hearing the furious beating of my heart, I think maybe I'm in the wrong profession. Maybe mommyhood is not for me. But even as the thought creeps through my mind, I know it cannot be true. I must be doing something wrong.

The next day I am lying in the solarium reading a book, and I find my answer.

"As desirable as contentment might be, however, it does not constitute happiness. Absence of a negative feeling does not constitute a positive feeling ... While being free of discontent may be fine for a cow, it does not suffice for a human being" (*Happiness and the Human Spirit*, Rabbi Twerski).

I think about all the times that I have been comfortable with – even grateful for – plain, ordinary contentment, but felt somehow as if something was missing. I read further: "Being the best we can be may vary with time and circumstances." I wonder, how can I be the best that I can be when I feel imprisoned in a role that feels too small for me? I feel guilty even as I think that.

Raising children isn't a trivial goal. Being a wife and a homemaker is praiseworthy. But why don't I feel it? Why do I feel more alive when I am running in an empty field or climbing rocks at dawn? Then God shows me the answer on the next page: "If we can do little but we do it wholly, we have a better chance at happiness than the person who can do much but instead does little." And the realization hits me right there in the silent solarium.

The same energy I use to reach the top of a mountain, I can use to listen to my child. The same way I can run until I am one with the wind, I can stretch my soul until I am one with His Will. Using the same mind I used to get an "A" on an Organic Chemistry exam, I can manage my household as if it's one of the Fortune 500 companies.

Why should my home, which in some ways will last forever, be run with less ambition and seriousness than a financial venture that will be gone in a century or less? For the first time in a long while I allow that voice to surface and ask the ancient question, "Is this what you got an Ivy League education for? To change diapers?" I let the question hang in the air for a moment, my book clutched in my hands and my white terry cloth robe wrapping me in a long forgotten cocoon of comfort. Then I find my voice. It whispers, "Yes. Yes. This is why God gave me an Ivy league education. This is why God made me a marathon runner."

This has never occurred to me before. I had always put my academic and athletic achievements into a different corner of my mind. Now I realize that this is a mistake. I can climb mountains while cooking dinner. I *can* cross the finish line in my own living room. All I have to do is focus and put my whole heart into whatever I am doing.

Later that night I sit in an over-stuffed armchair next to the brick fireplace and listen to a sixty-five-year-old woman speak about her life. When I tell her that I have several young children, she sighs and with a faraway look in her eyes whispers, "I wish I could go back and do that again." She speaks so softly and so wistfully I can hardly hear her. "Do what again?" I ask. She straightens her scarf and looks toward the window. "Raise my children again. I spent all those years wishing I was somewhere else and now that I'm somewhere else, I would give everything I have to go back and be a better mother. We wish away those years, only to beg for them back."

On the way home from the spa I stare out at the mountains that cradle our ascent to Jerusalem, and then I read one last precious nugget: "The measure of our happiness lies in our self-fulfillment, in being the best that we can be, even – maybe especially – in tough circumstances. Being able to analyze our present circumstances and develop 'a new yardstick' for the measurement of our value is the key to our pursuit of happiness."

I think about the marathon awaiting me in my home, and I begin to train my body and my mind to run the longest, most beautiful race I have ever run. I step out of the car into the noisy street, filled with the laughter of children, and I see a distant finish line weaving its way toward eternity.

*Originally published online at Aish.com, 2007.*

# BALM

*Tracy Thompson*

I have anxiety. Sometimes it's the worst part of this deal, this ongoing battle with depression. It's like a fire, smoldering in the brain, something wrong with the wiring that doesn't shut down the apparatus – oh no, it keeps working, if anything speeds it up – but impedes its function, gives it more to do than can possibly be done. And it feels, if this makes any sense, like a mental burn. You can't forget it for a second; it's with you always, like acid on exposed nerve endings. After a while, all you think about is relief. This is why people drink; it's why they do drugs.

So this morning I woke up and felt it descend again, this constant companion of mine, as I was getting ready to go to the gym. I thought swimming would help. Sometimes physical activity does help; sometimes exercise to the point of exhaustion is the only thing that will help. I was going to take my oldest daughter with me. We had the gym bag packed. She was downstairs, ready to go, and I was tidying up obsessively – making the bed, folding blankets, plumping pillows – because that is one of the things I do when I have this affliction. I feel the need to try to control every element of my environment – which of course I cannot do – but the more I fail, the more I feel compelled to try, and no, don't ask me to color with you, or listen to this knock-knock joke, don't you see the linens must be folded? But this time, for some reason, it was different. This time, something just snapped. I fell across the bed.

I cannot do this anymore, I thought.

That was it; for a moment, no other thought occurred. I rolled over on my side. My mind, which had stopped in the middle of its frantic busy-ness, began to pick up speed again, but slower. Fortunately, my husband and I had been watching the James Bond movie, *Casino Royale*, on DVD the night before, and that intricate plot became my next obsession, taking my mind off myself for a moment. I began to worry it, working out nuances, making connections, turning it over and over and gnawing on it like a dog with an old pork chop. After a while I became aware of the fact that I was getting cold, and I grabbed a blanket from the foot of the bed, covered myself, and lay down again. My mind slowed more. Outside I could hear the rain. I heard birds – at least three different kind of bird calls. I listened to the birds. I listened to the rain.

I said to the cosmos: Help.

All the while I was expecting my daughter to come bursting in, or my husband to trek upstairs to ask what in the world had happened to me, but nobody came. The house was quiet. I lay there some more, and slowly the mental burn subsided, and my mind's white-hot activity slowed some more. The birds were talking to the sky, to each other, and I lay there and listened. After a while, the rain picked up, and the drops fell faster and faster, and then, after some indeterminate period, I fell asleep.

And when I woke up, I felt – not healed, that was too much to expect, only fairytales work that way – but more whole. Calm. I went downstairs, and my family was there, and my husband said, "I thought you needed to sleep." My oldest daughter said, "Mom! I made finger sandwiches!" and my six-year-old came up to me and put her arms around my waist and said, "Mommy, snuggle."

And I said to the cosmos: Thank you.

# THE SPECTER OF DEATH, THE MEANING OF LIFE

*Laurie Henneman*

Having the specter of death hovering over my shoulder has helped me sort out my priorities in life.

I was thirty-nine when I was diagnosed with invasive breast cancer. I had just completed a postdoctoral fellowship in biology at the University of Montana and was about to start my first paying job in years. Instead, feeling completely healthy, I flew to Seattle and spent the next six months of my life getting chopped up and poisoned.

My daughter was two and a half at the time. The distraction of a toddler was useful in keeping our minds off the looming prognosis. Between doctor appointments and testing, we were able to take in the sights of Seattle, visit the aquarium, have lunch at the revolving restaurant atop the Space Needle, and see live fish at Pike Place Market. Through the eyes of a two-year-old, it was all a big, exciting adventure. She was delighted with the new experiences she had at hospitals, and while she understood in the months that followed that Mommy was "delicate," she was also thrilled by the novelty of my bald head and hospital beds that move back and forth. To this day, when we read *Curious George Goes to the Hospital,* she can't understand why the little girl Betsy is afraid to be at the hospital with George. To her, hospitals are interesting places full of fascinating devices and friendly people helping Mommy.

My daughter kept me busy and my family provided unwavering

support during my ordeal but, as anyone who has experienced cancer knows, the sickness is ultimately yours alone. After a bilateral mastectomy and a subsequent surgery to extract lymph nodes, I began six months of chemo hell. I became the "crazy woman in the attic," literally holing myself up in the third floor of our house while battling pain and debilitating fatigue. It helped me understand what my father meant when he described his first naval cruise: "First, you were so sick you were afraid you were going to die; then, you were so sick that you were afraid that you weren't."

I was given a drug to boost my white-blood-cell count, which left me feeling like my bones and organs were trying to turn themselves inside out. On top of this, I received the bonus prize of being one of the hapless two percent of patients who are allergic to one of the compounds I was being given, and so spent a tortured night covered with hives until they readjusted the drugs I was taking. I wanted to jump overboard, but I couldn't. I was committed for four months. Four long months.

Before I started chemo, I had been scheduled to teach a course at the university. Somehow, I clung to the hope that I could manage it. That was before I learned about "chemo-brain," a sometimes long-lasting condition in which the signals bouncing around up there start slogging through molasses. Incredibly, doctors refused to acknowledge chemo-brain as a real phenomenon until recently. Why exactly they found it so hard to believe that poisoning someone on a regular basis might negatively affect their most sensitive organ is beyond me, but they did. I limited my intellectual work to writing a blog for my friends and family to update them on my progress and . attempting to play a bit of the saxophone. My plans to teach were put on hold. If you ask most chemo patients, they'll probably tell you that the last treatment is the hardest to get over. The unpoisoned may not realize it, but there is a strong psychological component to withstanding the high doses of toxicity that permeate your body with each treatment. You hold on and bring yourself back before each hit because you have to. But when you know you've just had the last one, both body and soul tend to fall apart, and it takes much longer to recover. When I rang the bell at my oncologist's after my last treatment, I had no sense of triumph.

Two years have passed since my last treatment. I'm back to work on a number of freelance projects that allow me time to spend with my now five-year-old daughter. My priority now is my family and the privilege of watching my child grow up.  I know she'll emerge successfully into adulthood whether I'm here or not. But selfishly, I want to know her as an independent adult making her own way in the world. Every day, when I take my estrogen-inhibiting pill, I remind myself of how lucky I am to be alive. And while the specter of death remains, it hovers, thankfully, far back in the shadows.

# PART SIX

# THE STAY-AT-HOME STRUGGLE

೮೮೮೮

*It's not easy being a mother. If it were easy, fathers would do it.*

— The Golden Girls

# OBSERVATIONS FROM THE PLANET SAHM

*Sue Repko*

I am nothing if not a woman of action.

That's how I ended up sitting in front of a security guard at the entrance to an educational testing firm in central New Jersey – my husband's employer – in torn jeans and a stretched-out Ocean Pacific sweatshirt that had been on sale at T.J. Maxx four years earlier.

It was 8:10 a.m., and all the grownups were arriving for work, striding through the glass doors with their briefcases and the occasional mug of coffee. I tried making myself smaller, pulling my limbs in close. I averted my gaze and concentrated on constructing in my head a litany of curses against my husband, who was not at his desk. My shoulder-length red hair was still wet, and my bicycle was parked outside. I clutched a pair of black gloves and a ski mask. And then there were the slippers – extraordinarily pink and extraordinarily fluffy – that had also been on sale and which I'd given myself as a present from Santa, hoping to get a laugh out of my family.

Mission accomplished.

And now the rest of the world was in on the joke, too. Unless, of course, they had some glimmer of compassion for the mad woman – was she hearing voices? – huddled up in the corner.

Now, I'm not going to blame motherhood entirely for my impromptu clown performance.

Or my alienation from the professional world.

195

Or my anger at my husband.

Or my dance around the edges of insanity.

Well, maybe I am, because it was motherhood that created the conditions in which all these could flourish.

Back in the middle of February, 1991, I spent the night with my legs spread wide while virtual strangers came and went, free to peer and poke as they wished at the core of my very self, in a not-made-for-TV movie that I would call, The Demise of Dignity. At the end of that long, long night, when my firstborn – Alexander – was vacuumed out, I finally got a good look at the creature who had gradually taken over my body. How to fathom his very existence?

In a profound state of awe at the dawning of that new day, I packed up my ego and stored it in a cool, dry place, out of direct sunlight, where it would remain for the next eighteen years or so. Oh, it's gotten out a few times, to be sure. But whenever it seemed it might reassert itself, it ended up crawling back inside its little cocoon, back to life among the shadows.

I had stepped outside to wave goodbye to the men in my life: my husband and our two young sons. A wicked March wind stung my cheeks and whipped my wet hair into my eyes as they backed out of the garage and started on their morning commute. When I turned to go back inside, I realized that the shiny red door of our house was closed. And locked. I broke into an all-out sprint down the driveway, in my fuzzy pink slippers, waving and screaming. To no avail.

The car turned left and zipped down our country road. The three of them were gone, and I was left behind, locked outside my dwelling on the Planet of SAHM (Stay-At-Home-Moms). While this planet looks an awful lot like earth, the women there tend to exhibit a wide range of afflictions: sleek body syndrome, tidy home disease, progressive PTA disorder, and personality disintegration. In the common manifestation of the latter, a woman consistently refers to herself in the third person as "Mommy." Her "I" has gone AWOL.

In the most radical cases, a SAHM might suffer from all these maladies at once, and her life becomes a Sisyphean struggle to maintain body, home, children and community work, according to unimpeachable standards. These shimmering chimeras, with a drink in one hand and a glittering clutch in the other, appear regularly in the glossy pages of those local lifestyle/advertising magazines at some benefit or other, beacons to the rest of us. They really have their shit together.

If I were diagnosing myself, I'd say I suffer the most from a bad case of progressive PTA disorder, having taken on too many volunteer positions in my sons' schools and also in the communities where we've lived. But the diagnosis is complicated by the fact of my part-time employment sprinkled in over the years, activities that have given me the patina of having a "career," while not actually having one, and certainly not bringing in much money. After graduating from Princeton in 1984 with a degree in psychology, I eventually landed a job in Trenton for a federal housing program, certifying families' income and going in and out of dangerous neighborhoods, inspecting apartments. After a year, I went back to school to study urban planning and public policy at Rutgers University, one of the top programs in the country. I was named Planning Student of the Year and had my pick of jobs. At the tender age of twenty-six, I became the first housing manager for Princeton Township, a town that was progressively seeking to fulfill its state affordable housing mandate. Someone called me their "Housing Czarina." I had arrived.

Two years later, Alex was born, and all that professional momentum shifted. Although I'd come of age during the Women's Liberation Movement, the example of my own self-sacrificing mother of six had left an indelible imprint. After Alex's birth, I took off for twelve weeks, with a growing sense that I would never go back full-time. My employer did let me work part-time, but after a few months, I called it quits. I wanted to be at home, and I wanted to have another child.

I started writing for an affordable housing journal, my first freelancing gig, and did some consulting. It wasn't until after Jeffrey's birth in 1993 that I gave up on the idea of having an easily identifiable career. It seemed there was not enough space in my head to hear clear prose anymore; it was as though a switch had tripped. For a while, numbers and spreadsheets didn't make as much sense. When giving directions or reading a map, I became periodically

SAMANTHA PARENT WALRAVENS

dyslexic, mixing up left and right, east and west. What kind of planner did that?

On that morning of the pink slippers, the impetus that had carried me down the driveway now propelled me back to the garage. Maybe – just maybe – the broken phone in there would miraculously have a dial tone when I picked it up. No such luck.

I could not face any of our neighbors in my current condition. Most of our houses were set back from the road in the woods, and we were all relatively private people. It would have been too awkward to shuffle up to any of their doors in those slippers and then wait for who-knew-how-long, making small talk until Ken got to his desk, listened to his voicemail and drove back home. No, the only person whose help I would accept would be the same person who'd gotten me into this mess – Ken, of course. If only he'd heard or seen me earlier. If only he didn't drive so fast. He might have even been the one who forgot to turn the little button on the doorknob into the unlocked position. Now that I thought about it, he was also responsible for the way I was dressed. I might have taken a little more pride in my appearance if he didn't make so much money as a software engineer that it didn't make sense for me to go back to work.

He worked just two miles from our home, and I figured I could get there by bicycle just as he arrived. In the garage, I scared up a pair of gloves and one of the kids' black ski masks from the mini-van. I tucked in my hair and hit the road, pedaling fast to get the blood flowing as the wind brought tears to my eyes. About halfway there, I turned off our rural road and entered the flow of traffic on a county artery. Cars whizzed past. No doubt they held people Ken and I knew: respectable, normal people who would have no idea that the lunatic biking on that frigid morning was me. And I was grateful for the anonymity.

Childrearing is basically an anonymous endeavor. As mothers, we're locked inside our own private bubbles, and every once in a while our bubbles bounce gently into, and briefly join, other bubbles at the playground, in the supermarket or in the carpool lines. And then there are the once or twice yearly parent-teacher conferences –

which are really about the children's performances, but which Ken and I have always taken as measures of our parenting. Otherwise, it has felt like no one was really paying any attention to what I was "doing." From the mundane tasks of laundry and food prep to the higher-order demands of comforting the sick and seizing a teachable moment – these were all invisible to the outside world.

When the boys were about ten and twelve years old, I got it into my head that I should be paid for what I had surely earned all those years. How dare society not find a way to compensate its mothers? And as a planner, I believed in the power of grassroots organizing. In this case, a successful revolution would have to start at home, so I directed my lobbying efforts at Ken.

"I want you to pay me! I want you to acknowledge what I do! Every Friday, I want you to cut a check, made out to me! I almost don't care about the amount. Almost! But I want to get paid every week like real people who are doing something that someone else values. Like you. You get paid! I want to get paid. Someone has to pay me, and it's going to be you!"

He looked at me like I was insane. I vented some more. I cried. It blew over.

Well, not quite.

A few days later he handed me a scrap of paper.

"I took the Schwab account and split it right down the middle. This amount is now in your name. There's the account number. You can do what you want with it. Keep it in cash. Invest it. Spend it. And the other half of the account is still in both our names because what's mine is ours, and what's yours is yours."

Touché.

Well, that shut me up. Briefly. Because while I did appreciate having something in the bank to call my own, Ken's solution had gotten him off the hook from having to repeatedly thank me for being the incredibly wonderful mother of his children, which was a big part of the recognition I craved, all of which perhaps says more about our poor communication and nurturing skills with each other at the time than it says about society.

But such is the nature of long-married life. As of this writing,

SAMANTHA PARENT WALRAVENS

we've been together for twenty-five years. He has also sacrificed emotionally and physically to care for the kids. Bearing the entire financial burden of the household has taken its toll on him. He's ten years older than me but went prematurely gray a long time ago. He's had blood pressure and heart scares and panic attacks. Until recently, with the help of therapists, we tended to do what was expedient to solve an emotional problem. For a long time, we'd both sucked up bad feelings without airing them. And then there I was, having an emotional breakdown and demanding something that I'd never even mentioned before, something that didn't come naturally to either of us – praising the other for what had become the routine of our lives.

Since becoming a mother, I've been on a quest for some elusive balance. The recalibration never ends. If any woman thinks she's going to make only one decision – to work or not to work – she needs to think again. Because that's what she'll actually be doing – thinking, again and again. It's never been just an either/or proposition. There are always additional questions like, "what type of work?" and "how much?" Paid or unpaid, it's all still work.

Superwomen, beware: three or four part-time gigs can easily exceed the demands of one full-time gig. Trying to juggle multiple, unrelated tasks over the long-term can be detrimental to physical and mental wellbeing. It's pretty easy to keep piling on, to start that headlong tumble down the slippery slope of "yes" – oh, sure, I can fit that in – until you find yourself, a couple decades later, in a heap at the bottom of some hill, coming out of a coma, wondering, "How the hell did I get here?" Looking back, I wish I had not lost consciousness, that I had been more present, that I had let time pass of its own accord, rather than filling it up to hurry it along.

When my husband finally arrived at work that morning, I popped up from my chair to intercept him outside. He wheeled the bike back to the car. While he wedged the bike into the trunk, I sat stony-faced in the front seat. If anyone happened to recognize me now, they'd see my unyielding profile and know that nothing could break me, not even some dumb slippers.

But the truth is, those slippers were actually comfortable. Christmas was a distant memory. Their initial aesthetic assault on the eyes had faded. The joke was over, so what was the harm in wearing them around the house? It's the kind of thing a writer could get away with. Or a stay-at-home mom. By the time Ken unlocked the front door for me back at the house, we were both having a good laugh, and I kissed him and sent him on his way.

# KEEPING UP WITH THE FAMILY RIDE

*Abi Cotler O'Roarty*

I have this recurring image that I can't get out of my head. My husband is driving a car, maybe an old pickup truck, and I'm attached to a rope tied to the bumper. Whenever he steps on the gas, I go bouncing along faster and faster behind him.

It's not as bad as it sounds. Really. I don't associate any pain with the scenario – well, not physical pain anyhow. There is just a feeling that whenever that truck lurches forward, I go running madly, arms akimbo, trying to keep up.

When not conjuring up reckless scenarios, I am, among other things, a stay-at-home mom to two girls. My eight-month-old babbles a soundtrack of actual angels and grins like she swallowed a light bulb at the mere hint of her sister. Her sister, whom I would gladly have represent me in court, can argue at age three with the best of them, especially if the issue is someone telling her "no." I have to remind myself to hold firm in the face of her Shirley Temple curls and her calculating mind. Good thing she is also the most dedicated cuddler on the planet.

"I know how lucky I am to be home with them," I tell my husband when trying to approach the whole car bumper thing. I need him to understand how it feels to be in charge of the girls all day, the hours I toil with them defined solely by the hours he works outside the home.

My guilt at even approaching this topic begins to speak. "I know how special it is to get to soak up all their beauty and new discoveries every day," I add.

"And you know that when I'm not working toward a paycheck," he responds patiently, "I see it as a fifty-fifty deal all the way."

And I do know that. It's just the *not* in "not working" that gets me.

My husband's hours are messy and variable and you never know exactly what the workweek will bring. We spend many a Sunday night going over his upcoming schedule, our eyes already aching for bed – or at least some HBO.

And it can change at a moment's notice. Sometimes, just as I expect him to come home and help out with bedtimes, he calls to say, "The client needs us to tweak some things by morning, so I may be pulling an all-nighter." I think about the possible bed-wetting or teething baby in my future and think, *then so will I.* How quickly things can go from watching for his headlights in the driveway, fussy baby in arms, to hunkering down for the second shift.

Even last-minute travel is not off the board. And, of course, whenever he's crisscrossing Florida in a rental car for ten days, I'm at home putting the pedal to the metal, too. So, when he gets home from the airport, our girls have to witness their parents racing each other to the bed for a nap, throwing fouls with elbows all the way.

What gets me is the lack of any sense of control over how long I will work, or how hard. With over a decade in the workforce behind me, I am no stranger to hard work. But even on the most grueling day at the office, I could usually stop to get a cup of coffee when drowning in the muck of overworked exhaustion.

In my current career, this isn't usually so. The other day I left home for the market and just knew I couldn't make it through the trip without caffeine. But the stop for coffee proved to be a fatal error. The time it took me to do that was just enough to push the baby into her end-of-day witching hour, and the groceries ended up getting slammed into the cart, Baby screaming into my face from the carrier the whole time.

"At least you can go to the bathroom any time you want.... and in private" I tell him, in denial about how much my whine sounds like our three-year-old's. "I'm stuck trying to calculate the least bad time to sneak away, feeling like I'm back in school raising my hand for a hall pass." My husband, who knew me back when I used to get dressed in the mornings and jot down meetings in a neat little personal organizer, usually nods in sympathy.

Unless, of course, he does not. Unless he's exhausted, too, and hears my hall pass analogy as the opening play in the latest round of "Who's Got it Worse." Then he might remind me about the trip to the zoo we took last week while he lugged heavy equipment across a football field in the hot sun. To which I'll retort, "But I had to wear a shirt stained with poop on that trip 'cause the only person I don't pack extra clothes for is me." And the bell dings for another round.

Any married person worth her salt knows that when you begin to keep score, compare, compete with each other, you're on the fast track to the couch for the night. The same is true of getting too involved in the other's daily minutia. "Please, stop micromanaging me," he'll plead, and even though I know he's right, I just can't stop thinking that the three hours of work he's calling necessary on Saturday could be cut down to one if he'd only been more organized during the week.

Picking over my husband's efficacy at the office is the last thing I'd have thought I'd do before we had kids. It's right up there with begging him to eat lunch at his desk because I'm desperate to go alone to my doctor's appointment that afternoon. Before we had children, that kind of behavior would seem clingy, controlling and just not very fun. But the bond of co-parenting has a way of changing all that, and if I'm not careful, next thing I know I'll be going through his cell phone to make sure he took no personal calls at work that day. I mean, when you're still in your bathrobe at 5 p.m., what's just one more step toward crazy?

When I confess my dark, car-bumper image to fellow stay-at-home moms, many nod in recognition. Sitting on a grassy hill at the playground, one tells me of her anger at her professor husband for announcing that now that his book is published – a book which consumed his entire summer *off* – it was time to follow it up while the iron was still hot. "Instead of being happy at his success and cheering him on," she admits, "I found myself livid that he would even consider it."

Another, whose partner often travels on business, offers the question, "What if when they asked, no *told* him, he had to fly to Pittsburgh next time, he said he didn't have anyone to watch his children? That'd make them think," she says, jolly at the thought.

It's true. Does the workplace just assume the stay-at-home parent is signed up to stay home interminably? Are we the stay-at-home-all-the-time parent? What of our needs? Our time off? But I should know better than to ask about time off in today's Blackberry climate of sixty-hour workweeks. Perhaps this is another symptom of American worship of industry above all else?

Tonight I finally brought up the bumper thing with Ian and, understandably, he balked. "Do you think I'm really in the driver's seat?" he said. "Don't you think I'd like to not pull an all-nighter or say 'no' to traveling once in a while?"

And I know he's right. The pressure he is under to take care of us all on his single salary is great. He's on a formidable treadmill of his own.

Re-enter the guilt. Supersized.

There is so much privilege that comes with this package, too. I'm incredibly grateful to be the one there, to guide my kids so consistently as they first wake up to the world. And I get so much more of the fun stuff than he does, running private jokes with a baby and a preschooler, getting to teach small fingers to pinch pie dough just as my mother did when I was young.

So maybe my husband is not driving the car, after all. But he's in the passenger seat, at least. And if I'm not getting dragged behind the bumper, I do still see my skirt caught in the door as I try to get out.

# IS NEVER GOOD FOR YOU?

*Shannon Hyland-Tassava*

It's happening again. Just home from preschool pick-up, I'm scrambling about the kitchen in a mad dash to put lunch on the table before my two- and four-year-old girls dissolve into a puddle of pre-nap, hunger-fueled tears. The microwave is beeping, my toddler is tracking boot-slush throughout the entryway, and my oldest is regaling me with a tale of nursery-school social dynamics when the phone rings, barely audible over the lunchtime din. I check the caller ID and smack my forehead. It's an old grad-school friend from Chicago, calling from her office, hoping, no doubt, to catch up. Though I love this friend dearly and owe her more than one well-intentioned phone call, I quickly mute the ringer and rescue the peas from the microwave, the baby from her snow-caked boots, and the preschooler, who is now on the potty calling for help from her bathroom predicament – "Mama, I need help WIPING!" Catching up with an old friend will have to wait. About three to five years, I'd guess.

Later on, my friend sends me an email that reads, "I just tried to call you at home so we could chat. Let me know when would be a good time to talk!" I dash off a quick reply between quelling the baby's naptime rebellion and tending to the odd bit of freelance-consulting work that I occasionally field during my daughters' naps: "Sorry about that; I couldn't pick up!" I write. "A good time to talk would be …" and then I successfully fight the urge to type "never."

I wasn't always like this. I'm a relationship-driven nurturer at heart, and before having kids, my friendships meant everything to me. True, I was never the most devoted lover of the telephone, and I've always tended toward the introverted end of the social spectrum, but long-winded evening heart-to-hearts or lazy weekend coffee dates with the various members of my small but cherished group of dearest friends were a regular part of my routine. I excelled at email contact and (pre-electronic-age) letter-writing. I was the one who reached out, caught up, kept meticulously in touch with old friends from high school, college, previous jobs. I was never a social butterfly, but if you were my friend, I wanted to hear from you on a regular basis. I wanted to spend my free time, or at least some of it, talking to you.

But that was before I lost all my free time.

I'm a mother now, and an at-home mother at that. As a stay-at-home mom to two children under five, my time is rarely my own. Gone are the days of freewheeling social planning, of phone conversations – or even just a sentence! – uninterrupted by baby shrieks and toddler squeals. While rewarding and, in my eyes, worth every sacrifice, this job of full-time mothering is jam-packed and nonstop: days filled to the brim with diaper changes, sippy-cup spills, preschool runs and laundry loads. Half the time I'm simultaneously trying to cook dinner, schedule the pediatrician appointment, and referee a battle over who gets the pink Play-Doh, all without losing my mind. I don't usually have time to worry about losing my friends.

But I'm not like this with everyone. My local fellow at-home-mom friends and I keep up a steady stream of social contact, supporting one another on a daily basis through the challenges of tantrums, toilet training, and time-outs. But our conversations are clipped, unfinished – a mad dash of one-line emails and prematurely-ended phone calls, peppered with disruptions by our kids – and we're comfortable with that. We're in tune with the rhythms of one another's days, with each other's time limits and more pressing priorities, because they're ours as well. We stay connected in fits and starts over the sounds of toddler music class, during the breaks at library story-time. We don't call at lunchtime, because we know there's no time to talk then; we're too busy.

It's not that I don't think my working-mom (or working non-

208

parent) friends are busy, too. I know they're all juggling jobs, social commitments, and family demands just like I am. But I also remember my days as an office-bound professional, and recall that those days, unlike my current ones, included things like lunch hours, coffee breaks, and the occasional aimless afternoon spent surfing the Internet or catching up on personal phone calls. These days, the only thing aimless about my at-home-mom afternoons is my to-do list, which keeps getting interrupted by the patter and chatter of toddler feet and mouths. I wake up each morning to the urgent call of diaper-changing and milk-pouring, and most days I don't even get a solo bathroom visit, let alone a lunch break that involves attention to my personal needs rather than the feeding of other people.

When my husband relieves me from childcare duty at the end of his office workday, there's dinner to prepare. At the end of the day, when the children are tucked into bed and I've completed both my regular five-mile run and a post-workout shower, I've got approximately an hour of free time before I fall into bed in my pursuit of a solid eight hours before my early-rising girls begin a new day. When weighing the options of devoting that hour to a long-overdue phone call with a far-away friend versus collapsing on the couch in front of *The Office* with a bowl of Ben & Jerry's, dessert and TV generally win out. After all, it's the only "me-time" I get.

I guess I assume that this phase of minimal me-time will eventually pass, and, with it, my difficulty balancing family and friends, solo and social endeavors. I envision a future stage of kids in school, perhaps a return to the world of offices and lunch breaks, hours free of the constant physical needs of very young children. I imagine that then I will have the time and energy to include regular long-distance phone calls to old friends in my calendar, to plan visits, to willingly – and with pleasure – give up an evening hour of couch-time and cable for a drink with a long-lost girlfriend, an unhurried conversation with a former classmate. I can only hope my working-girl friends will wait for me.

In the meantime, I don't apologize for needing my scant hours of unscheduled time to recharge my own batteries with solitary pursuits, even if those pursuits include nothing more than chocolate and the latest issue of *People* magazine. It's what I need to get by, these days. And a true friend understands.

# CONFESSIONS OF A CRAZY MOMMY

*Darcy Mayers*

Tonight I ran away from home.

I shoved my husband's keys in my purse along with two beers, and I took off. I had nowhere to go, but if I stayed at home any longer, it might have gotten worse.

I don't need to tell you what started the ordeal. Let's leave it at: kids piss off parents. Let's leave the details about who did what and why and when to whom to your own imagination.

After all, I am not confessing that my kids can be headstrong and fiendish at times. They are kids, after all. I am confessing to the quality of my reaction – ugly and bad. Maybe it's some latent religious instinct that makes me think that if I tell the story, I can live better with it.

First, I yelled. I collared two kids and sent them to their rooms. One fled. One didn't. I yelled again, a close-the-windows kind of loud. She talked back, lingered and made excuses.

When she got mouthy again, I stood up from my stool and lunged. I lunged like a bear for blood. Startled, she burst into tears. I said or maybe snarled, "You better be scared" and then I chased her up the stairs. I picked up a lousy sweater at the threshold of her room and I snapped it her way. I am not sure if it hit her; I was blind with rage and frustration and I felt like I could throw her out the window.

But I didn't. I ran downstairs, out of breath and panting and literally shaking with adrenaline and guilt and anger and horror about what I had just done. Then I puked in the kitchen sink.

That's when I grabbed my coat and the car keys and the beers and took off. I told my husband the tenderloin would ding when it was done.

After I was halfway down the street, panting more than breathing, I pulled the car over. I called my high school roommate – who only just moved to town from another country and who has two very little kids and a very big job and travels a lot – and she didn't answer. I went to her house anyway, even though I wasn't totally sure where it was and even though I knew their furniture hadn't yet arrived and that it was Monday. At 7:30 p.m.

I was fully prepared to just sit on their front steps, like a sad hobo, and breathe for a minute before sulking home. Instead, they welcomed my sobby, puffy face into their own regular mayhem.

She knew just by looking at me that I wasn't there to chat. She hustled me up to their bedroom and let me burst into tears. She listened and nodded and wiped a couple drops off my cheeks. I started to feel amazed at how long we had known each other and how many tears we had swiped off each others' cheeks and how it was kind of stunning that here we were again, not fifteen anymore, but here together and I was crying about something that was really bad.

*I ran away from home*, I cried and confessed. I laid out my sorry stay-at-home mom tale for a savvy international business woman who took in my hobo self and bolstered it and loved it back to okay.

I drove home later that night knowing again that I am not the woman my college diploma says I am. I drove home to the house with the naughty, loudmouth kids who are not my career or my job and not my diploma and not even me. I drove to the house I live in and make mistakes in and in which every decent thing I love lives.

Do not judge what I did.

I scared my child and I wanted her to be scared and I puked in the kitchen sink.

# ARE YOU FAT, OR JUST PREGNANT?

*Amy Schneider*

I was the only woman at a table of twenty in the private dining room of a fancy restaurant. Some people already had their top-shelf vodka drinks, and the expensive wine was starting to flow. At least three courses were coming, not including the port and coffee at the end. The whole thing would cost more than an average family of four takes home in a month. All in all, it was a typical team dinner for my consulting company. I was part of a large group working with our client to create and implement a new software system that would run the core of their business. It was a huge project and a large team. Out of the twenty-five people from my company working on the project, two were women – a younger, single girl (she wasn't there that night) and me.

This dinner was shaping up to be one of those four-hour deals, tedious under the best of circumstances. I had put in my usual twelve hours of work that day, and I now had to sit and make small talk when all I wanted to do was to go back to my hotel, watch *Sex and the City*, and catch up on personal email. But I sat gamely chitchatting, sipping on my drink.

About halfway through, the guy to my right turned to me and said – as if he was just making conversation – "So does your husband mind that you're so fat?"

Oh yes, I was eight months' pregnant.

I really couldn't tell you what my response was. I was so

flabbergasted that I think I just sat there with my mouth open. The reaction from the couple of guys – both senior to me – who heard was immediate but … unsatisfactory. I think they punched the idiot and told me I looked great. And that was it. I dropped it. I regret a little not bringing it up to the partner the next day – just so he could talk to the Idiot and impress upon him that he had dodged a bullet because I'm so cool. What I mean is, if the Idiot had said that to a more litigious, sensitive woman, the company could have a real problem. But I had a little thing about being "the cool one." The one girl in double-accelerated math in middle school with a bunch of boys. The only girl in the programming class. The only girl in the IT department. I liked being one of the guys. Being pregnant – tough to be one of the guys.

The type of consulting I did was right up my alley. Talk about "one of the guys" – not many women get MBAs, even fewer specialize in the intersection of business and technology. It was also a one-hundred-percent travel job. You left on Monday morning at the crack of dawn and got on a plane to go to your client's offices, wherever they might be. On Thursday or Friday night, you flew home. This schedule, of course, becomes a grind. But when you're single (or at least in the "I'm focusing on my job" mode), it's pretty glamorous. I flew first class all the time, stayed in fancy hotels, ate at the best restaurants. You know those lists in airplane magazines of the best steakhouses in the country? I've been to most of them. The people who have a special key to the executive floor of a hotel? That was me. On some flights I even got to make my own ice cream sundaes. Not a bad way to travel.

The other thing about consulting that suited me was the "up or out" culture. Your performance was reviewed rigorously every six months, both on its own merits and against everyone else at your level. Each level was force-ranked and the bottom ten percent was axed. This system did not scare me. I liked the competition. I had always gotten the top grades in school and best performance ratings in other jobs. I was good at what I did and slowly built a reputation for being someone who gets things done.

During my time with the firm, I went from being totally single to dating someone exclusively, getting engaged, and getting married. A year after our wedding, my husband and I decided to start trying to have a baby, not an easy task for someone who is on the road four nights a week. Then an opportunity came up that allowed me to work from home for a few months. In typical goal-oriented fashion, I was determined to make this baby happen during this period. Check.

Just a few weeks after becoming pregnant, I developed crushing nausea: 24/7, debilitating morning sickness, right as I was going back on the road. I was staffed on a project in Chicago (flying in from Connecticut) with about five other consultants. We were one of several groups helping to design and implement a new software system. Soon after starting the assignment, I was sitting in a conference room at the client's offices with two guys on the team, going over a project plan I had written. It was going slowly. A wave of nausea overcame me and I realized I had to make a quick exit to avoid heaving all over the conference table. I hadn't told anyone I was pregnant yet, much less work people. Besides the usual "anything could happen" reason, to be pregnant in my world seemed … weak.

If I didn't eat constantly, I would vomit. And in that meeting, despite snacking on crackers and Coke, I knew I had lost the battle. I rushed from the conference room to the bathroom as fast as I could. Now, the good thing about being a female consultant working on a floor filled with programmers and other consultants is that the women's bathroom is usually deserted. I threw up and then lay on the floor, too weak to get up and soothed by the cold tile.

I dragged myself, white as a sheet no doubt, into the partner's office and explained I was sick and had to go back to the hotel. The partner was a great guy with four children of his own. He probably guessed what was going on but kindly accepted my explanation. I think we both would have been appalled had he delved further. Back at my fancy hotel I called down to room service and asked for "dry scrambled eggs, white toast, a coke, a ginger ale, and saltines. Charge me whatever you want."

Naturally I cut it a little close. Just one week after getting "off the road," I had our daughter. In three years I hadn't slept at home for more than four consecutive nights, and here I was at home, a first time mother with a tiny baby depending on me for her very life. I was terrified.

All of my life I had been "career-oriented." I played "Company" with my dad's briefcase when I was a kid. I liked working and was good at what I did, but my job was 24/7 and consumed all my energy. The travel requirements were such that I would only see my baby on weekends. My husband and I decided together that I would quit and stay home.

Giving up the money (more than half our family income) was hard. Giving up the label and the prestige was harder. Transitioning from working to not working is a huge adjustment for anybody, and for me it was almost a 180. I thrived on the imposed structure of office hours and meetings and deadlines. I liked the "grades" and feedback. Without a job, I had to make my own structure, subject to the caprice of a difficult baby. No one was there to tell me how I was doing. Feeding her and getting her to sleep were victories. But where was the "A" I was used to getting, and where was my bonus?

I decided that being a mom was my job now, and that I should approach it that way. I labeled myself the "Household Manager," with job responsibilities including grocery shopping, cooking, cleaning, laundry, picture-taking, corresponding with relatives, buying Christmas presents, challenging insurance bills, hemming pants, getting the oil changed, and more. All those "things" big and small have to get done by somebody. In my new job, I was in charge of everything.

Household Manager. Hmm. This description made sense to me but lacked the bit of glamour I was used to in my previous job. When I was working, I was unique in being a techy, business-oriented woman. Now I was just another stay-at-home mom, struggling with the relentlessness of my job. The trouble with motherhood and household work is that they are constant, but despite all your work, you never seem to get ahead. The minute you feel a sense of accomplishment, you have to do it all over again just hours later. "The baby took a great nap this afternoon!" Oops, now we need to get her to sleep again three hours later. "The living room is dusted and vacuumed!" Oops, now there are cracker crumbs all over the floor. "Dinner was delicious, used up the leftovers, and the kitchen is clean!" Oops, we're out of milk for breakfast tomorrow.

For someone who needs to stay on top of everything and feel in-control and organized, the inability to "get ahead" in my mom job can be crushing. When I got behind at work or had a deadline approaching, I could go in early, work late, rearrange things, focus, and knock it out. Staying home with children, this focus is just not possible. Your time increments to concentrate on anything and get any project accomplished shrink. And by "project" I mean anything from painting the bathroom to writing an email to a college friend who's having a tough time. Instead of working 8:00 p.m. to 11:00 p.m. to finish a presentation, let's say, you have three fifteen-minute increments from 7 a.m. to 5 p.m., plus, if you're lucky, one-and-a-half hours at nap time. And you still have to get the minimum of your "daily jobs" done (feeding everyone) before doing a project. You can forget the night – it's the only time that you have to spend alone with your husband, even if you're just falling asleep in front of the TV together. This inability to control my own schedule and focus and accomplish anything is the single biggest adjustment – really ongoing struggle – of staying home.

Even after doing this job for four years – now with two children – I chafe sometimes at the constant demands and attention that small children require. Then I feel guilty for being annoyed. Remember going to the pool or the beach when you were little and the few times that your mom would get in the water and play with you? Remember how thrilling that was when she did? I do. I want to be the mom who plays in the pool. But I'm also the mom who finds it impossible to leave a task half done.

It's a battle I fight constantly. On the one hand, I don't want my kids to think that this whole family exists for their entertainment. I want them to know that daily life takes work and that, for the most part, Daddy and I do most of it for them now, but when they are older they will contribute. Laundry does not magically get clean and land in their drawer; a special wind does not come up and blow the leaves off the lawn. Being part of a family entails responsibility and involvement. On the other hand, my daughter needs me to participate in the fantasy world she's constructed to make it operate as she has pictured. My son wants me to whisk him around the hall in a laundry basket. I want to be a participant in their world, but I also want to exist in mine.

I've resisted reading the Mommy blogs and joining Mommy groups. I am deathly afraid of Facebook. I think I'm trying to ensure that I'm not identified as "just" a mom. Which is weird because I think that being just a mom – um, Household Manager – is wonderful. I think that being primarily responsible for turning a helpless infant into an ethical, smart, kind person is laughably undervalued, actually. Still, there's probably a little chip on my shoulder that's discernible to others in Mom-world. I don't stand out any more.

When I quit to stay home, I always thought – and told myself – there would be an "and":

"I stay home … and I do freelance PowerPoint work on the side."

"I stay home … and tutor the neighborhood kids in math."

"I stay home … and write novels."

Something. What I didn't realize is the mental and physical toll that motherhood takes on you. I envisioned myself getting up at 5 a.m. to write or work on something personal. What a crock! I know the story goes that JK Rowling wrote Harry Potter at the café with a baby in the stroller. But who was doing her grocery shopping and vacuuming her living room and cooking her dinners? And how do I get a baby who will sleep in a stroller for a couple of hours? Mine did not. Thanks JK for making us all feel bad about ourselves.

There's no "and" for me. The alarming thing is, I'm not sure if there ever will be. Am I a consultant who took a break to get her children "up and running"? Am I a mom bringing her business skills to bear on running a household? Am I an entrepreneur who will take all of her business and Mom-world knowledge and use it to create something great? I have no idea. That's the problem. I'm trying to be all those things in a misguided effort not to be "just a mom" – when what I should be doing is existing in the moment with my kids and my husband and myself. Though it has served me well, I feel I need to tamp down my end-goal-seeking personality and revel in how lucky I am.

Though sometimes I struggle, I do not regret my decision to stay home. I know the investment will pay off for me, for my children, even for my husband, both in ways I can see and in ways I can't possibly fathom. My degrees, my experience, and my ambition are still in my back pocket. For now, I use them in service to my family. I can mimic an expensive party invitation in PowerPoint; plan and pack for a week at the beach down to the last detail; create an analysis of prices in area grocery stores; perform tech support and training for grandparents. And, lest I forget, teach my kids how to read, add, share, apologize, learn, travel, plan, be on time, and be a good friend.

I'm not sure if I'll ever be good enough for me, but I'd like to think I'm good enough for them.

# THE PRO MOM

*Darcy Mayers*

This is what I have learned so far about the world of children: it is tiny and enormous. There are bugs more interesting than great books, and questions about heaven and happiness that would puzzle even the greatest philosophers. It's all or nothing, and also all and nothing. It changes daily. You learn to go with it.

This is what I have learned about motherhood, stay-at-home motherhood: it's a jungle in here. As it was in the office, so it is behind the picket fence. Talk around the office cooler is now playground chitchat. The company picnic is now the PTA meeting. The geography has changed, but the jockeying and one-upmanship remain the same. I didn't realize when I left my career to stay home with my kids that I would be facing a different but even fiercer form of competition: competitive mothering.

It wasn't long after I became a full-time mom that I came face to face with my nemesis: the Professional Career Woman Turned Mother. To keep it simple, I'll just refer to her as the "Pro Mom." You know her. She is one of the millions of women who benefited from every wave of feminism. She picked a job she wanted, and she succeeded: doctor, lawyer, banker, teacher, consultant. Maybe because she could do it all, or because she wanted so badly to do it all, she became a mom. Unable to keep up the pace at work and at home, she gave up her career for the kids. Like I did.

Having quit a lucrative career to stay home, the Pro Mom takes her mothering responsibilities very seriously. She engages her newborn in sign language, music classes, and potty training before he can sit up. She considers co-sleeping, attachment parenting, and nursing-on-demand not an option, but a requisite. She relishes a Baby Bjorn culture that glues the baby to the body. When the kids hit school age, there's Spanish and French, team gymnastics, travel soccer, tennis, baseball, painting, ice hockey and lacrosse.

Even on the days when I've whipped up homemade play dough or read my child the same book six times in a row, I know the Pro Mom is out there, outdoing me. She is tapping endlessly into her Blackberry the schedules of her accelerated children, reminding me that no matter what I do, I am not doing enough.

As women, we have brought this culture of competitive mothering onto ourselves. When I was in college, the smart, feminist girls like myself waged a minor rebellion – one of many that stood to pit us against old-school feministas. It was okay to be sexy, we said, to like men, and to wear mascara and short skirts. We viewed our sexuality as a tool and not a limitation. Marriage was okay, as was motherhood. We would have it all – finally! We would have respect and hot pants and all the babies we wanted and promotions that paid for our cute new shoes. We supported each other, hired each other, built businesses together, formed women's networks, and made changes.

So why is it that when we make the biggest decision of our lives – to have children – the camaraderie of our earlier feminist experiences suddenly backfires? Why is it that our powerful girls' network dwindles to a homemade dinner dropped at the front door when a new baby arrives? Maybe it's the distance from the shackles of our past, or the comfort of our modern success, but in the moment of our most feminine experience – motherhood – we forget what has given us the possibility of becoming super women in the first place: each other.

The world remains tiny and enormous. Children ask a million questions because, as it turns out, there are that many. There is more than one answer. You don't need to be a Pro Mom to know that.

# THE PINK POST-IT UMBRELLA

*Devorah Lifshutz*

On the morning that it happened, the news reported that a Missouri man opened fire at a city council meeting and killed eight people. Glancing at the headline, I felt a twinge of smugness, albeit tinged with shame.

Look, I told myself, proof that you aren't the craziest person on the planet – that there is someone else out there who's got soul storms that rage wilder than your own. I needed to remember that, because of my own internal attack of heavy weather. Unlike the Missouri man's, my tempest brought forth no damage unless you include the scars on the souls of my young son and myself.

The morning followed a pattern that seemed to be hardening into a template. The script was quite ordinary – just me struggling to get Danny, my eight-year-old son, out to the school bus, but somehow today our combined personalities, emotions and reactions crashed against each other in a giant thunderclap.

As I sat at my kitchen table doing postmortem on my outburst, I couldn't figure it out. Why did I lose it? I was an experienced mom, a full-time stay-at-home. Danny was the fourth of five kids. I knew this territory: getting kids out in the morning, making their lunches, getting them onto their buses.

In my better moments, I could see that Danny was a beautiful boy with straight brown hair that fell upon his forehead in a fringe, a little genius who brought home perfect report cards and could add

223

and subtract long columns in his head.

But then there was this other Danny, the Danny who, on this particular morning, had nearly driven me insane.

I played back the morning in my mind. The wake-up had gone well, normal, the usual way. I'd tiptoed into his bedroom, bent over his ear, whispering my own little wakeup song: "Time to get up, time to get up, time to get up," I sang over and over in a bouncy, melodic voice. He knew the song. He could even harmonize to it if he wanted to.

His eyes still shut, Danny took my hand into his and grasped it close. For a few minutes, I sat beside him on the bed as rays of dim winter sunshine streamed in through the window behind us. But the morning was rolling along. I reminded Danny to get up, laid out his clothes for him. He dressed and showed up for breakfast right on time. A good omen, I told myself tentatively. On other mornings, Danny would just linger in under the covers until I'd dress him and rush him out the door.

This morning I had Cocoa Pops, his favorite. No brownie points for nutrition, I thought, though the package insisted that they contained fiber and vitamins.

"No," he said rubbing his eyes, and turning his head away from the bright yellow box.

"C'mon," I nudged. "It's important to eat."

No response. Danny just sat in the kitchen chair, his head hanging down. He looked like someone on an airplane, trying to sleep sitting up.

I'd seen this before, this morning freeze-up. Maddening, having one's kid go on the blink like that without any reason. Unlike on my laptop, there wasn't anything to click or press to get him started. In my mind, I'd come to call this eight-year-old catatonia. Usually it went on for a few minutes, but then he'd wake up, get his coat on, and get to the bus. Today the re-emergence was taking too long.

"C'mon, it's getting late," I said, an edginess creeping into my voice. Still no answer.

According to the oversized kitchen clock, there were ten minutes left until the bus arrived, which felt like ten minutes to blast-off or ten minutes to doomsday. I was crazy with this – making sure that Danny got his little body onto the bus.

"What do you want for snack today?" I asked, hoping the promise of a snack would rouse him from his seated slumber.

"Pretzels," he mumbled, chewing the word with his breath.

I reached up into the cabinet. "No pretzels. How about cookies?" I offered, trying to paint over my tension with a saccharine voice.

"NO," Danny yelled. "IF I DON'T GET THE PRETZELS, THEN I'M NOT GOING TO SCHOOL!!!"

Danny slipped back in catatonia, just sitting, staring at nothing at all, thinking, I suppose, about pretzels – sticks, rounds, pretzel shapes, even honeycomb patterns these days, pretzel coatings, salt or sesame, whole wheat or white?

Meanwhile, I was losing it … fast.

I glanced up at the clock. "It's time to go." Silence. "Now!" I yelled, as if the increased vocal volume might cause the neurotransmitters in his brain to respond.

Danny did get up, but instead of going out the front door with his back pack and parka, he ran into the living room and landed on the couch.

"Danny, come here," I said, lowering my tone a few octaves to sound like a general or a drill sergeant, at the very least.

Danny started running wild circles round our long dining room table.

"Come here," I commanded. He refused to stop. I was now officially furious. My mind flashed to my neighbor Judy, half my age with nearly as many kids – how her son, Davy, two years Danny's junior, was getting what Judy defined as "a little wild," grabbing his sisters Legos, a misdemeanor in my book, and how Judy sent him into time-out without even elevating her tone one decibel. I could never get Danny to do that. I couldn't get Danny to listen to me at all. Maybe it was Danny, I thought. He was defective, like Rosemary's Baby or Damian, one of those monster kids you see in horror movies. Meanwhile Danny was circling faster and faster, and my fury was hitting new peaks.

"You little s---," I yelled, shocked that I had used a word that was forbidden in our house. I picked up one of his favorite toys, a Playmobil fire truck, and smashed it against the hard ceramic tiled floor, causing the wheels to fly off the chassis. For a split second Danny stopped, frozen in place. I pushed the table toward him, sandwiching his body between the wall and the table. He was trapped, nabbed, captured. Then I lunged toward him, bracing my hands around the soft bones in his neck. For one very long second I thought of pressing hard, just squeezing the breath out of him. How easy that would be. His bones were still so soft, almost like chicken bones, but then I stopped myself. Lowering my grasp and anchoring my hands under his arm, I lifted him and his jacket and his backpack outside to the bus stop.

My mind was still on that bus – making that bus – as if that would somehow redeem the morning. As we stood together outside in the cold February morning, my anger came spilling out in hard, painful words.

"Why do you do this to me? Are you crazy? Do you want to make me crazy?"

Danny burst into tears, sweet little boy tears. Suddenly I loved him again. He was my son, sweet Danny. I drew close to hug him, but he pushed me away. What did I expect? Then the bus honked. Danny ran outside and got on sullenly, without looking back. That was it. For a long time, I stood at the bus stop, just staring out into space. My job was done. He made the bus, but this small victory did nothing to lift my spirits or undo any damage I had done to my young boy's psyche.

As I turned back into the house, terrible questions racked my brain.

Was I really like that man in Missouri – capable of wild violence? Was I a child abuser? Was I inflicting permanent damage on my son? Was I unfit to be a mother?

I felt numb, paralyzed. I really didn't have a good answer, just a lot of bad feelings I would have loved to erase. Maybe I could just pretend, I told myself, start all over, make-believe this hadn't happened. Give Danny a big smile, prepare his favorite lunch when he got home and hope he just forgot. Yes, yes, feigned amnesia. Part of me was pleased with that idea, but my great big superego conscience that had left me during those terrible moments not so long ago suddenly found its voice.

No, you can't just make-believe. You've got to use this, to move forward, to do it better the next time.

An old Jewish teaching popped up in my head – something I'd heard a million times, almost a cliché. *A righteous person falls seven times and gets up.* What did that mean? That a righteous person was a jack-in-the-box or one of those bloodied prize fighters?

Now suddenly the words made sense. The righteous person lost it, maybe even big-time. He messed up, screwed up, but he went back and tried again and again and again. Over and over, up and down. That was the process of life. And that was what made him righteous.

That was my job now, too, to get myself up again. To rise up above this morning and make sure it never happened this way again. I grabbed a black pilot marker and started writing: "Mommy's Rising Plan," I called it.

"Mommy's Rules." Not for Danny, but for me. On a hot-pink Post-it square I wrote them down:

> No cursing.
> No throwing things.
> No calling children "crazy."
> No strangling.
> If the child doesn't cooperate, just wait and do nothing!

The rules were for me, to grab hold of, to remind me that even when things were at their craziest, I was the mommy and I had to keep a handle on myself. Besides, I had tools and leverage, lots of it. I could give and take away life, but I could also give and take away videos, play dates, Game Boy cartridges, Cheetos and Doritos, even the spicy ones. I stuck the Post-its all over the place, on the fridge, on the front door, on my bedroom door, on the mirror, in my closet – everywhere. It didn't matter that Danny would read them or anyone else for that matter. I needed them to grab on to when my anger threatened to carry me away. They were my little pink paper umbrellas, my shelter for the next storm.

**Author's Note:** As it turned out, the pink Post-it umbrella was not the elixir I was hoping for. A few months and many tantrums later, Danny took a hammer to his MP3 player and smashed it. At my wit's end, I took him for an evaluation with a neuro-psychologist who, after six hours of testing, diagnosed him with ADD (without the H) and something called "Attachment Disorder," which I later discovered was on the autistic spectrum. At first I freaked out, blaming myself for my son's problems. What "attachment disorder" means, however, is that something is missing in my son's psyche; the glue that should bind him to mother, to parents and to himself is in short supply. Through counseling, we are learning to build up Danny's glue supply. Our therapist has taught us to be a lot gentler with Danny, who though chronologically a fourth grader, is emotionally still in nursery school. For his part, Danny seems happier and easier to live with. By the way, I don't use the school bus anymore. Extravagant as it sounds, I send Danny to school by taxi. He can sleep a half hour longer and arrive at school feeling calm and relaxed. Both he and I are happier for it.

# GENTLY USED

*Katherine Ozment*

It took forty-five minutes from the time I placed the ad on Craigslist – "Free couch to anyone who wants it!" – for two young women to show up in our parking space behind our house and haul it away. I was loading sippy cups into the dishwasher when I heard their voices, and I peered out the window to see two twenty-somethings in shorts and t-shirts heaving the overstuffed white hulk of a sleeper sofa into the back of their SUV.

That couch had been with me for ten years and six moves around the country. When I described it in the ad as "gently used," I wasn't quite telling the truth. I'd bought it when I was twenty-eight, a single working woman living in Washington, D.C. It was my first real purchase, bought in the heady days just after I had landed a promotion from researcher to full-fledged editor at *National Geographic* magazine. I had spent many nights curled up on that couch, jotting notes in the margins of manuscripts. Later, my husband and I shared our first kiss on that couch. And, when he was offered a post-doc at UC-Berkeley and I decided to jettison my job and follow him away from everything I knew, we hired a man from the Want Ads to cart it down the tight stairwell of my apartment building and put it on a truck bound for California.

As my husband's academic career took off and I started and quit several jobs, we hauled the couch from Berkeley to Chicago and then to Boston. I nursed our son through nights of colic on that couch, and when our daughter was born and I gave up working outside the home, I spent hours with her on the sofa, teaching her Pat-A-Cake, getting her dressed, and folding what sometimes seemed like hundreds of tiny shirts and onesies.

Last week, I watched the couch make its final, ungraceful descent down a flight of stairs as the men who had delivered our son's new bunk bed took it out to the curb. I was determined to get it picked up before night came with its forecast of rain, so I rushed to the computer, logged on to Craigslist, and searched for words to describe it, settling on "very comfortable," "attractive," and "gently used." None could embody everything that the couch had meant to me, but my main mission was to get rid of it. After my quick success, I felt a combination of triumph and longing for the person I'd been, back when I had first bought it.

Through the years of moving and motherhood, I've let my career fall by the wayside. I no longer work as a journalist or even in an office. I don't have a business card or a boss. I'm now a part-time freelance writer, working between childcare drop-offs and pick-ups in my jeans at a desk in our basement, rising intermittently to wash a load of clothes, marinate a pound of chicken, or haul out the trash. In any given year, I earn enough to buy myself an occasional sweater. I am, I reluctantly admit, a member of the "Opt-Out Revolution," a place I've come to in steps, some so huge I fretted over them for months and some so small I didn't even notice myself taking them.

I'd be lying if I said I didn't miss my old life. I miss the clear-cut trade of work hours for a paycheck. I miss black pantsuits and shoes that click when I walk. I miss riding the bus each morning with my coffee, newspaper, and sense of genuine purpose. And the hush that would come over the room on the ninth floor at *National Geographic* headquarters when a photographer just back from Sierra Leone or Borneo would flash breathtaking images from the field onto the screen before us, and I would sense that I was part of something much bigger than myself.

Mostly, I miss the ambition I saw in those young women after they'd wrestled their prize into their truck and tied it down. It was the way they got in and drove off with the urgency of people who have somewhere to get to and the freedom of people who have no one to take care of but themselves that made me catch my breath.

At thirty-nine, I'm starting to understand that life has seasons, and mine is nearing the end of summer. What concerns me now are things like how to calm the anxiety brimming in my son's eyes or whether my daughter will grow up with a positive body image.

Where my heart used to leap at a travel assignment to a faraway place or a positive review from my boss, I now find joy in moments no one else sees: striding behind my son as he wobbles down the sidewalk on his first bike ride to school or watching my daughter wrap her mouth around the word "spider" for the first time. It's then that the label "Opt-Out" seems all wrong to me. In truth, I feel more "in" my life than ever, connected to a purpose – the love and care of my children – that is pure in a way no job I ever had was.

And yet, as I watched the couch disappear down our street, I couldn't help but feel a little jealous of those women, perched at the outset of their adult lives and careers. I wondered: Who are they? What do they do? What will they tell their friends about their great find?

"Can you believe it?" they might say. "We saw the ad on Craigslist and got there first!"

I wish now that I'd gone outside to talk to them before they left. But what would I have said? That you have to press the metal crossbar down hard so the bed doesn't bump up in the middle. That the feet need new scuff pads. That the small punctures on the arms are from our cats and the stain on that one pillow is just apple juice. Is there anything I know that they might not figure out on their own?

Maybe.

I would have told them to enjoy it.

*Originally published in Skirt! magazine, March 2008.*

# REGRETS OF A STAY-AT-HOME MOM

## *by Katy Read*

We had wonderful times together, my sons and I. The parks. The beaches. The swing set moments when I would realize, watching the boys swoop back and forth, that someday these afternoons would seem to have rushed past in nanoseconds, and I would pause, mid-push, to savor the experience while it lasted.

Now I lie awake at 3 a.m., terrified that as a result I am permanently financially screwed.

As of my divorce last year, I'm the single mother of two almost-men whose taste for playgrounds has been replaced by one for high-end consumer products and who will be, in a few more nanoseconds, ready for college. My income – freelance writing, child support, a couple of menial part-time jobs – doesn't cover my current expenses, let alone my retirement or the kids' tuition. It is a truth universally acknowledged that a single woman in possession of two teenagers must be in want of a steady paycheck and employer-sponsored health insurance.

My attempt to find work could hardly be more ill-timed, with unemployment near 10 percent, with the newspaper industry that once employed me seemingly going the way of blacksmithing. And though I have tried to scrub age-revealing details from my résumé, let's just say my work history is long enough to be a liability, making me simultaneously overqualified and underqualified.

But my biggest handicap may be my history of spending daylight hours in the company of my own kids.

Just having them is bad enough. Research shows that mothers earn 4 to 15 percent less than non-mothers with comparable jobs and qualifications, that as job candidates, mothers are perceived as less competent and committed than non-mothers (fathers, in contrast, rate higher than men without kids). Heather Boushey, senior economist at the Center for American Progress, told me last year that the outlook for an at-home mother returning to work in this economy "kind of makes my stomach drop a little bit." I know the feeling.

When Paul Krugman warns that many of the currently jobless "will never work again," I am petrified – hello, 3 a.m.! – that he means me. I long ago lost track of how many jobs I have applied for, including some I wouldn't have looked twice at in my twenties, but I can count the resulting interviews and have fingers left to twiddle idly. Before I left full-time work in 1996, my then-husband and I, both reporters at the same newspaper, earned the exact same salary. Now my ex, still a reporter, is making $30,000 a year more than that, while I have been passed over for jobs paying $20,000 less.

As I wander the ghost-town job boards, e-mailing my résumé into oblivion, I tamp down panic with soothing thoughts: I have a comfortable house, for now, some money in the bank, for now, a nine-year-old Mazda that rattles alarmingly but runs, for now. Millions of people are hanging by far thinner threads, and I am genuinely grateful for what good fortune I have.

So this is not a plea for sympathy. More like a warning from the front lines.

The recession has already shifted habits and attitudes and will likely usher in long-term cultural changes about which economists, sociologists and political strategists are churning out predictions as we speak. Here's mine: The economic crisis will erode women's interest in "opting out" to care for children, heightening awareness that giving up financial independence – quitting work altogether or even, as I did, going part-time – leaves one frighteningly vulnerable. However emotionally rewarding it may be for all involved, staying home with children exacts a serious, enduring vocational toll that largely explains the lingering pay gap between men and women as well as women's higher rate of poverty. With the recession having raised the stakes, fewer mothers may be willing to take the risk. If it's not yet the twilight of the stay-at-home mother, it could be her late afternoon. Certainly it is long past nap time.

Statistics suggest mothers are reaching that conclusion. Between 2008 and 2010, the number of stay-at-home mothers fell from 5.3 million to 5 million. (Stay-at-home dads held steady at around 150,000.) Who knows how many others are frantically sending out résumés? Whether they have paying jobs or not, mothers still handle most of the country's child care, but that "feels like the last gasp of a dying age," journalist Hanna Rosin wrote last year in *Atlantic Monthly*. She quotes Boushey, noting that "the idealized family – he works, she stays home – hardly exists anymore." The image of a mother pushing a stroller down the street at midday may come to seem as quaint as that of a 1950s housewife pushing a vacuum in stockings and pumps.

Stay-at-home mothers obsolete? Those among the 5 million who are alive and well and reading this may have something to say about that. Go ahead and vent, stay-at-home mothers. I get it. Fourteen years ago, I struggled with my own decision amid a tangle of internal and external messages. Some still seem valid and others now less so, but the difference was hard to tell amid the hormone-saturated, sleep-deprived, advice-swamped bewilderment of new parenthood.

I became a mother during a moment in history when women faced unprecedented career opportunities yet were expected to maintain a level of interaction with their children that would have made my own mother's eyes roll practically out of their sockets. I was a busy reporter and naive new mom – two jobs that I was led to believe could not, for all practical purposes, be performed adequately and simultaneously. Oh, and while one was commendable, the other was morally imperative.

Like I needed the extra pressure. I already felt responsible for giving my sons childhoods – those fleeting years that would forever loom large in their lives – full of adventure and learning and treasured memories. If I could have enriched their experience by moving to a farm or hitting the road in an Airstream, I would have considered it. But according to the parenting manuals I dutifully consulted, what my boys required was constant engagement with a loving, omnipresent figure, sort of like if God engaged in daily floor time. The parenting experts never said exactly how children like mine, overseen by an ever-shifting cast of underpaid near-strangers in a commercial daycare center, would be damaged. But I got the impression I might as well have gone through pregnancy throwing back shots of tequila.

Meanwhile, my work/life balance ... wasn't. My husband and I kept erratic hours, handing off babies like batons. At work, I lost choice assignments as I dashed out before the stroke of 6, when the daycare began charging a dollar a minute. My editors, probably well-meaning, set me on what suspiciously resembled a mommy track. While an intern handled the tragic late-breaking news of an honor student murdered by her mother's crack dealer, I yawned through meetings where citizens complained about potholes. (Though who knew how fabulous a steady-paying pothole gig would look to my underemployed future self?)

And the emotional turbulence! I drove to work with spit-up-stained shirt and tear-streaked face, cried at baby-food commercials featuring mothers and infants bonding in what looked like a weekday-afternoon glow. I felt the time flying past. My firstborn wasn't yet crawling when I began gazing nostalgically at newborns in the park, with their impossibly delicate fingers and mewing cries. Over at the playground, hulking four-year-olds hoisted themselves around with huge, capable hands, conversing in vast vocabularies. Soon my son would be one of these giants, his infancy vanished into the chaotic past.

My second son was born. Two weeks later, my father was diagnosed with a brain tumor. Sitting near my dad's bedside, I showed off the baby to my Aunt Millicent, mentioning my plans to return to my job. She shook her head sadly.

"You won't believe how fast those years go by," my aunt said. "Try not to miss them, if you can help it."

My father died two months later. That fall, my husband found a new job in a different city. And I – feminist, ambitious journalist, daughter of a woman with a successful advertising career – quit a full-time job at a big-city paper and began part-time freelancing work that brought in less, some years, than I'd made as a waitress in college.

I wasn't worried, frankly, about the long-term economic consequences, partly because nobody else seemed to be. Most articles and books about what came to be called "opting out" focused on the budgeting challenges of dropping to one paycheck – belt-tightening measures shared by both parents – while barely touching on the longer-term sacrifices borne primarily by the parent who quits: the lost promotions, raises and retirement benefits; the atrophied skills and frayed professional networks. The difficulty of reentering the workforce after years away was underreported, the ramifications of divorce, widowhood or a partner's layoff hardly considered. It was as though at-home mothers could count on being financially supported happily ever after, as though a permanent and fully employed spouse were the new Prince Charming.

I myself witlessly contributed to the misinformation when I wrote an article about opting out for a now-defunct personal-finance magazine. Amid chirpy budgeting tips and tales of middle-class couples cheerfully scraping by, I quoted a financial advisor bluntly outlining the long-term risks. My editor wasn't pleased. "It's so … negative," she said, and over the phone I could almost hear her nose wrinkling. So I, neophyte freelancer eager to accommodate well-paying client, turned in a rewrite with a more positive spin.

Since then, a few writers have reported the financial downsides, notably Ann Crittenden, who calculated in "The Price of Motherhood" (2001) that having a child costs the average college-educated woman more than a million dollars in lifetime income. More recently , Linda Hirshman ("Get to Work," 2006) and Leslie Bennetts ("The Feminine Mistake," 2007) wrote manifestos scolding women who opt out. In 2010, Karine Moe and Dianna Shandy outlined the risks of downsizing a career on behalf of family in "Glass Ceilings & 100-Hour Couples."

But I might not have realized such warnings even applied to me:

After all, I was working. Downsizing my career seemed ideal – research shows 60 percent of mothers would choose part-time work if they could. While my kids spent three afternoons a week in daycare, I did what the experts advised: developed my skills, undertook new challenges, expanded my professional contacts. I advanced creatively if not financially, published essays in respected literary journals that often paid (cue ominous music) in copies of the magazine.

But who had time for long-term financial planning amid the daily demands of two small boys? I took them sliding, skating, swimming and skateboarding, supervised art projects, helped with homework, conferred with teachers, drove to music lessons and dentist appointments and baseball practices. I handled all of their sick days, some involving lingering health problems that, if I'd had an office job, would have exasperated the most flexible employer. Not every moment, of course, was sunny and delightful; there was plenty of crying, screaming and slamming doors (sometimes by the kids, too, ha ha). It was harder than any paying job I've ever held.

Salary experts estimate the market value of a stay-at-home parent's labor (child care, housecleaning, cooking, laundry, driving, etc.) at about $118,000. This hollowly cheerful calculation has always struck me as patronizing, with the effect, if not the intention, of further diminishing our status. Moms – aren't they the greatest? They should be pocketing as much as a registered pharmacist or the mayor of Chula Vista, California, yet they'll happily accept payment in the form of adorable gap-toothed smiles. An implied, faintly sinister coercion – a good mom doesn't want money – fuels a system that relies on our unpaid childcare, household chores and volunteer work but offers no safety net.

Few of the arguments for staying home seem as persuasive now as they did 14 years ago. I long ago stopped trusting most advice from so-called parenting experts. The kids I know who attended full-time daycare seem fine, and I doubt my sons would have been damaged if I had kept my job. In at least one crucial way, they'd be far better off: I'd have more money to contribute to their college educations.

Still, like most mothers, I have mixed feelings about my choices, and like most mothers writing complaining first-person essays, I feel compelled to note the upside. I am deeply thankful to have witnessed as much of my sons' childhoods as I did. I'm a procrastinator, and I can imagine myself thinking of those long playground afternoons as something I would get around to eventually, not noticing the swing set's shadow stretching ever longer across the sand.

So if some young woman with a new baby were to ask me about opting out, I would tell her, as my Aunt Millicent told me 14 years ago, how quickly a child's early years zip past, how challenging but wonderful they are, how grateful I am for every single moment I was privileged to witness.

And then, unlike my aunt, I would warn her not to do it.

*Originally published on Salon.com, January 2011*

# PART SEVEN

# MAYBE, BABY

ભજભજભજ

*Women have more options than in the past to build strong careers and to exercise the choice not to have children.*

– D'Vera Cohn, Census Bureau's
Population Survey 2010

# BIRTH MARK

*Deborah Fryer*

1 988 – The labor comes on fast without warning. The pain jolts me awake. There is no moon, so it's darker than usual. It must be after midnight. I am terrified. I am not supposed to be pregnant. I'm a first-year graduate student at Princeton, and I'm married to my books. I don't have a boyfriend. I can't even remember the last time I had sex.

I grip my down comforter tightly around my shoulders even though I'm dripping with sweat. I lie on my back, trying to calm myself, but my breath is ragged. I squeeze my eyes so hard, I'm seeing colors and sparkly lights. I can feel my books – standing row upon row like soldiers at attention – mocking me. Throughout my years as a student of the classics, I had counted on Vergil and Homer to protect me, on Horace to show me the middle path, on Euripides to teach me right from wrong. Now, in my moment of need, these old friends stand mute on their shelves, glowering in disappointed silence. I feel so ashamed.

There is a blur of people in blue smocks. Their faces stare down at me with concern. Someone adjusts an IV pole and jabs a needle into my arm. Another places my feet in stirrups. A third drapes my legs with a heavy cloth. The lights are blinding.

"Push, honey, push." The nurse's kind, brown eyes look into mine, but she is on the far end of a telescope. I can see her lips moving, but her voice comes out spongy and muffled like an echo across a wide valley. "You're doing great," she encourages me. "That's good, honey. I'm right here." She speaks in a Southern

243

drawl, dripping with honey. I squeeze her hand hard. I am afraid I might break her fingers.

Her eyes are my anchor. I lock onto them, and I push. And I push. If this storm gets any fiercer, I will surely be ripped apart. And then, suddenly, I am in the eye of the hurricane and all is quiet. There is wetness everywhere, and I feel the warm stickiness of my baby slithering out, all slippery and soft and long. The pain is gone and I am throbbing down there and tears are streaming down my cheeks. It's over. I'm done. At the nurse's urging, I find strength to push once more, and then the whole room inhales at once. There is a collective holding of breath. I can see from their faces that something is not quite right.

"What? What is it?" I cry. They are shaking their heads. Their hands cup over their gaping mouths and their eyes lurch in their heads like jack-o'-lanterns. "What's the matter?" I am hoarse. I am exhausted. I can barely get the words out, "Is it a boy or a girl?"

"Neither." The nurse extricates her fingers from mine. She shakes her head side to side in disbelief, and covers her mouth as though she is going to be sick.

"It's a Standard Poodle," she says, still shaking her head. "Lord have mercy."

When I open my eyes, sunlight is streaming through the curtains and the birds are singing. It is time to get up and get to class.

\* \* \*

1989 – I'm in Manhattan, in a starchy blue gown, underwearless, wearing paper slippers. My stomach is in knots. Sweat beads on my upper lip like a tribal tattoo. I feel like I might vomit at any moment. My breasts are damp with sweat, my elbows sticky. I wish I could wake up from this bad dream, but this time, it's real. I've created this nightmare, and it's all my fault. I should have been more careful.

The fluorescent lights in the elevator buzz like a swarm of angry hornets as I rise to the eleventh floor of a nondescript but very important-looking building on 32nd and Park. The waiting room is immaculate. The shiny hardwood floors wink in complicity, while the picture windows look the other way, down at the diamond-encrusted, Botox-stiffened women sauntering along the colonnaded avenue in their minks and Manolo Blahniks. I wonder if these wealthy wrinkle-free white women have any idea what's going on right over their noses, because it's clear up here that fertility snubs its nose at race and class.

"Debby," the receptionist calls.

"It's Deborah, please," I correct her. She hands me a cup to pee in and points me to the bathroom. "You know what to do," she says curtly. I fight back tears. I am on a hormonal roller coaster, and everything sets me off these days. In the bathroom, after I fill the cup, I splash cold water on my face and neck and let it drip down my chest. The coolness calms me. I'm going to go through with it. I'm so close to finishing my dissertation, I can't jump ship now, and I don't want to. I don't want to have a child. Not now. I'm not ready to be a mother, not to mention a single parent. I am not even sure who the father is. I thought I could compartmentalize, have serial boyfriends, be intimate with both, serious about neither. I thought I could color inside the lines. I was wrong. So now I wait here alone and ashamed, but clear that termination is the only option.

Every bone in my body aches. My skin feels filleted. My heart pummels me from the inside out. It's beating so hard, my chest hurts. Even my hair hurts. I have never felt so sad in my life.

There is a knock on the door. "Are you okay in there?" the nurse calls through the door. "Do you need some help?"

"I'm all right," I answer. My eyes are puffy, and I can't stop crying. I don't care. Once the spigot has been turned on, I can't shut it off. Tears rain down my cheeks and I don't even bother to wipe them away.

An Hispanic woman takes my medical history and $290 of my precious stipend; an Asian woman takes my blood, then leads me to the next room where two other accidentally pregnant women, equally doleful and draped in blue gowns, are waiting. A counselor describes the procedure we are all about to have. Do I want to be awake or asleep, she asks. I don't know. I have never done this before. Is it going to hurt? Chrisantia, an African-American woman to my right, starts sobbing. The counselor hands her a Kleenex, which she blows into loudly. Ruth, also African-American, is more composed and decisive. "This is not my first abortion," she proclaims with authority, "I definitely want to be put completely out." She jabs the air emphatically with her long red fingernails. Her gold hoop earrings nod in enthusiastic affirmation. She catches Chrisantia's eyes. "Take the meds, girlfriend," she advises. "Okay," Chrisantia sniffles.

But I decide that I want to be awake. I deserve to suffer. I deserve to experience all the pain and anguish and more. I was unconscious in my relationships with two men who loved me, I betrayed them both, and I feel so sick I think I'm going to throw up last night's Chinese food right there in the pre-op holding area. "I'll stay awake," I can barely get the words out. I'm so dizzy, it's all I can do to stay upright. "Awake." the counselor scribbles on my chart. "Awake?" Ruth raises an eyebrow. "You'll be sorry." I'm sorry I acted so unconsciously over the summer, I'm thinking. I don't want to be unconscious ever again. I clutch the armrest of the chair for support.

A nurse takes my elbow and guides me to the sonogram room, where she instructs me to lie down on a mint green table covered with paper. I stare at the ceiling and will it to stop spinning. She squirts some K-Y jelly on a plum tomato-shaped wand and presses it below my belly button. It's cold and ticklish. I try not to move. "You're too gaseous," she says. "I'm trying to see your uterus, but I can't see anything." She removes the tomato from my stomach and reaches for another instrument. This one looks like a curling iron. She globs more K-Y on the end and covers it with a condom. If only I had been using condoms a few months ago, I wouldn't be here. If only I hadn't … she guides that thing inside me and starts wiggling it around until there's a picture on her screen: a small white boomerang-shaped fetus swirling in its own little galaxy. She estimates that I am seven weeks pregnant. Do I want a picture of my baby? No, I do not. I want to erase this, want to delete this experience from my memory. The tears roll down the corners of my eyes and drip onto the paper-covered pillow. "I'm sorry, honey," she says, patting my arm, and helping me to sit up. "It's gonna be okay."

I pad in my paper slippers over to the next room, where they will .do the deed. A blonde nurse pushes her bangs over her plastic-rimmed glasses so she can see to take my temperature. Another nurse straps my legs in stirrups that are covered with potholders decorated with cherries. I appreciate that someone has been kind enough to create a soft barrier between the cold, hard metal of the stirrup and my bare skin. An African-American anesthesiologist comes to stand next to me. His nametag says George. I notice through his beard that his front teeth are chipped. "I'm just going to give you some fluids," he says, painlessly inserting a needle into my right arm and clamping a pulse oxymeter onto my index finger. "And I'm going to hold your hand. You just squeeze me if it hurts." His fingers are huge, his palm is warm and thick. My little hand disappears in his big one. "You squeeze as hard as you need to," he says."I'll be right here."

Dr. Black walks in, pale and young. He's all business. He pulls the mask over his bearded mouth and lowers the clear plastic glasses over his blue eyes. He wipes between my legs with a cold wet cloth. In one quick movement, he inserts the speculum, clicks it open, stabs a needle into my cervix, and then pulls everything out again. I breathe a sigh of relief. It's over, I think. That was no worse than a pap smear. But I'm wrong. "That was the local anesthetic," he says. "Scalpel, please."

He starts scraping. I squeeze George's hand. I remember when I lived on a Greek island and we sacrificed a lamb for Easter. I held the lamb's legs down while someone else slit her throat. She bleated bloodcurdling arpeggios as she bled out, trembling, fighting death, resisting with all her might. And then she relaxed into it. I heard her anguished cries but there was nothing I could do. This was the age-old ritual on the island, and I had chosen to step into ancient history. The plaintive cries lacerate my heart, and I recognize that wailing voice as my own. The doctor turns on a vacuum cleaner. I fight against the leg straps. I feel pulling, stretching, tearing, wrenching inside. I'm being ripped inside out. "Keep squeezing!" says the kind doctor whose hand I am still gripping. I look at our hands intertwined. I have turned his dark chocolate hand milk white.

The vacuum mercifully stops. The noise and the pain recede like a wave returning to the ocean, pulling the sand away from the shore. A blonde nurse comes to the head of the bed and wraps her cool hands against my cheeks. And then the scraping starts again. Three times, the doctor scrapes and vacuums. By the end of the ordeal, every nurse in the room is touching me, stroking my arms, my legs, comforting me, praising me for being so strong and still. And then it is silent. The doctor puts down his instruments and leaves the room. The procedure is over. But now cramps set in that are so intense I think I am beginning to die. The pain hits so hard, it takes away my voice. Somebody gives me an injection to make my uterus contract and I am wheeled into the recovery room.

There are about twenty women in the room, all waking up from general anesthesia. They moan and vomit into kidney-shaped plastic bowls, clutching their stomachs. Or they sleep like they are dead, with the whites of their eyes showing. When they wake, it's fitful; they toss and turn, puke, belch bile, lie back down again with a thud. I am glad that I chose to forgo the anesthesia. This looks much worse than what I went through. I feel sad and crampy, but at least I am not sick. At least I am all here, fully present, fully aware and awake. The worst is behind me, I think, dumped in a medical waste bucket. But deep down I know that the worst part lies ahead in the pain of recognition that I threw away two kind, good men who loved me, whom I loved, but not well enough.

In the post-recovery room I drink a bottle of water and eat a sugar cookie. It's dry and tasteless. I am bleeding copiously into a sanitary napkin as big as the Oxford Latin Dictionary. I want to go home.

For weeks I have cramps and constipation. My face breaks out. My hair turns brittle. I dress in nice clothes, try to trick myself into happiness, into normalcy, but in my heart I feel like I have fallen through the ice. Neither of my boyfriends wants anything to do with me anymore. Who could blame them? I want nothing to do with me, either, but I am stuck with me and my recklessness.

I deal the only way I know how. I work out like a maniac, train for a marathon, and start baking bread. I throw myself into my studies. Vergil and Homer protect me from my darkest self. Horace shows me the middle path, Euripides teaches me right from wrong. The poetry is all so beautiful, it cracks my heart open and lets in a ray of hope. Translating Greek and Latin is hard for me. I love the mystery of the puzzle, the dance between form and meaning, the challenge of making sense of something so ancient yet timelessly relevant. I love the musty smell of my books and the crinkly pages of my dictionary and the epiphany of clarity and understanding that comes eventually if I stare at the page long enough.

* * *

1999 – I'm walking through Midway Airport on a layover when I see the sign: ORCHIDS, it reads, in colorful, curly letters, TERMINAL B. I have time to kill, so I head over and find an actual greenhouse, right there in the middle of the airport, filled with intoxicatingly beautiful flowers: petals of fuchsia, violet and lemon chiffon curl like sensuous tongues around the stamens that drip with nectar. The leaves are plump, pulsating with wetness from the fine mist that hangs in the air. The smell makes me swoon. The beauty is almost too much to take in. I have to sit down.

A few minutes collapse into hours, and I realize that I am about to miss my flight. I sprint for the gate, running as fast as I can, but I know I'm not going to make it. I hear the announcement for last boarding call, and I run faster. I see the heavy jet-way door swing closed at the gate. I watch the red flashing lights over the door change from NOW BOARDING to PLANE DEPARTED.

My travel alarm beeps insistently. I open my eyes, and I don't know where I am. All hotel rooms look the same in the dark. Ever since I finished my PhD six years ago, and traded the stillness of the ivory tower for the fast-paced world of producing documentaries for public television, my life has been in perpetual motion. I'm lying disoriented, trying to figure out if I am in my own apartment or in Turkey or Tel Aviv, Mexico City or Selma, Alabama, when it hits me. My mind is still reeling from racing in my dream, but I lie still and let the truth sink in. It lands with a sickening thud. I know where I am. I am at a critical juncture in my life, and I need to pay attention. I have been here before – unconscious of the consequences of my actions until it's too late. Now I've divorced my books, and married my work. I'm still single, and 35, and my biological clock is ticking. I need to wake up, not for work. For my future.

My body tells me that this dream I just had was not about orchids. I feel that same constriction in my gut that I felt at Princeton. Back then, it was fear about having a child. This morning, it's the fear that it's already too late. My inner voice speaks the truth: this dream is about your choice to pursue a career as a filmmaker ... instead of having kids. Get it, she says? It was a visual pun. Orchids? Or kids? You were in a place of transition, an airport – an "heir" port. You chose to follow the beauty, the exoticism, to linger in the sensuality of experience, and then you missed your plane. You were running for it, but you didn't make it. If you want to have kids, you better get on it. Yes, I will get on it, I think, I will, I must.

But when?

The phone rings. It's my boss. Where am I? she wants to know. Our crew is already downstairs having breakfast, and we are leaving for our film shoot in fifteen minutes. I'll be right down, I promise. I stop thinking about the big picture of my life, and jump into the shower to get on with what I love at this moment.

* * *

2010 – I had always believed I would fall in love in my twenties, have children in my thirties, and be a tenured professor at some Ivy League school in my forties. But that plan was simply naïve and romantic, and as it turned out, the three fates – serendipity, chemistry and biology – had something completely different in store for me.

I met my husband shortly after my forty-second birthday. By then, the window of my fertility was coming to a close, along with my desire to have a child. For years we clung to the idea that if it happened, it was meant to be. And if it didn't happen, we would be fine with that, too. I was still menstruating regularly, and I could predict when my cycle would start down to the hour. Sometimes I could feel myself ovulate, and then I was sure that this time surely we were going to conceive.

When I was younger, I remember feeling relief every month when my period came. I didn't want to be pregnant until I was married, until I had established a career. I had endless time, I thought. I will know when I am ready, and I hadn't been ready. Now, I am ready, we are ready, but my body is no longer so eager. Now, I feel sadness each month when that small, irretrievable part of me detaches and flushes away.

A few months ago, my period was uncharacteristically late. I was filled with equal parts trepidation and exhilaration. Was it possible to get pregnant at age forty-six? Could I carry a healthy baby to term at this age? Would we have the energy to be good parents? Did we even *want* to be parents anymore? We had all but given up. My breasts became tender. I needed to sleep with the windows open, had to pee all the time. I obsessed over everything. By the end of the seventh week, I was having terrible cramps, and I knew something was wrong. These cramps were as bad as the ones I had felt twenty-two years earlier when I squeezed George's hand white. My husband and I decided that if the cramps didn't go away over the weekend, we'd call a doctor on Monday morning. Late that Sunday night, I felt the pressure release, and then blood poured out of me, and I delivered a human apostrophe into the toilet bowl. I stared at it, stunned, that tiny final contraction swirling in its own galaxy, silently punctuating an emptiness.

# EMPTY BELLY

*Majka Burhardt*

I was twenty days into a trip in northwestern Namibia when I stopped being able to answer my own questions about motherhood. It was early evening in the Marienfluss valley – that hour-long slice of time when the whitened grasslands are momentarily gold. I stood in the shadow of a granite face I'd just climbed, surrounded by a Himba family outside of their mud and grass home. I had no common language with the Himba, but they'd been watching my team rock-climb, and we'd been living on their land. One woman had a baby on her back, and she and I developed a system of pointing and gesturing that seemed the most efficient way to transmit information.

After we confirmed that we'd been climbing and they'd been watching, we switched to communicating about life. Her baby – six or eight months, I guessed – and I were making faces at each other. She turned to give me better access to the little boy, and when she moved sideways in the light I saw her round belly pushing against the orange and yellow blanket that covered her bare body below. I looked up at her and then together our eyes traveled back to her stomach. Within a moment she'd grabbed my hands and pulled them close. She flicked the woolen blanket out of the way with her elbow and settled my palms on the skin of her stomach. We kept them there until her baby kicked.

I thought we were done, but the woman wanted to touch my stomach next. Her right hand turned to a fist as she drew close to my navel, and when she touched me, her knuckles brushed my skin as if

253

knocking on a door. She rapped. Twice. She pointed at the rock face above. She shook her head, rapped again. "No, no, no," she said.

I'm a professional rock climber and climbing guide. For a decade and a half, starting in college, I have earned my living in conjunction with adventure. This has always been my dream. When I took the first step down this path I never expected that it would land me in a complicated conversation with myself about children.

I climb rocks, mountains, icefalls, any or all of it. I travel the world to do it, write about it, come home, move my home, and go again. Over the years, I have modified how much risk I take in these endeavors. In the world of climbing, I suppose one could argue that my life is much less risky than it once was. Outside of the climbing community, however, the fact that I lost a dozen friends in the mountains over an eighteen-month period last year makes my perception of relative risk moot. And it gets more complicated. The men I seem wired to love are also climbers and guides. They pursue the same things I do, sometimes with even more fire. Deep down, I suspect two things about them: that they might get killed, and that they won't make much money.

I am a feminist at heart. When I was young, I used to beat up kids who said "mankind." I'd have push-up contests with anyone within five years of my age. And I received the most roughing penalties in my fifth grade co-ed floor hockey league. I was tough, but I also wanted to have eight kids, all with names that rhymed.

Like all young women who grew up in the '70s and '80s, I was told that I could accomplish anything I wanted. I went into adulthood never questioning how living my dreams would intersect my plans for motherhood.

Now I'm thirty-four. Each additional year that I live my life the way I do – climbing, traveling, taking risks – I hear more and more people tell me they can't imagine me having children. It would be easy to agree with them and point to my career choice as an explanation of why I won't have kids. But the truth is much more complicated.

I would have children if I didn't have to change so much. It would be much more convenient if the man I love would change: if he could make good money, pursue a career that didn't put him in constant danger, tolerate my career volatility, and accept the risks I take. Then I would have children with him. There are so many things wrong about this vision. First, I never expected to have a partner who would support me and our family. I've always felt that providing for children should be a shared responsibility. Second, I understand that I do not have stability in my current lifestyle, but, secretly, that is exactly what I want the person closest to me to ooze.

I was not taught as a child how to live the life I am living now. Nor did I learn from others in this profession in high school, college, or graduate school. I grew up around people of action – people with ambition and resources who lived their dreams through established jobs with consistent paychecks. They risked their lives in ordinary ways like driving, eating too much red meat, and rollerblading without a helmet. Now I'm part of a generation who have directed their ambitions toward goals far less tangible. I want the same things that come with a conventional upbringing; I'm just trying to get them differently. I realize that my methods might not work.

In Namibia, I walked away from the pregnant Himba woman wishing I could talk to her about my inner conflict. But I didn't have the language to even start a conversation and I could barely explain my feelings to myself. I lay awake in my tent for a long time that night. My partner, who lay beside me, had fallen asleep as I told him that I could still feel the heat of the woman's belly in my hands. He is a man I might have children with. He is a man I might choose to love without children. What did I want? What did the woman want for me? What did my belly being empty mean to her? To me?

I stared up through the mesh screen at the stars in the southern hemisphere. I have never been good with stars. But that night, I worked on a new answer to the question of children and motherhood: I told myself I would have children if the constellations in my life were right. I know the coordinates I need to link – climbing, mobility, writing, adventure, love, communication, and a partner to share my life with. Maybe I will find them together. Maybe I won't.

# CONTRIBUTORS

**Kathryn Beaumont** is a journalist-turned-teacher-turned-a handful of other things-turned-attorney/writer. After receiving a bachelor's in English from Princeton University and a master's in journalism from the Columbia University Graduate School of Journalism, she worked as a journalist for publications such as the *Idaho Mountain Express*, *People Magazine*, *Technology Review*, and *BusinessWeek*. She has taught high school English and worked in higher education administration and, finally, attended Boston College Law School. She now practices law in Boston and lives just outside the city with her husband and two young children.

**Tara F. Bishop**, MD, is an Assistant Professor of Public Health and Medicine at Weill Cornell Medical School in New York City. She earned her BS degree in Chemical Engineering from the Massachusetts Institute of Technology and her MD degree from Weill Cornell Medical Center. Dr. Bishop took time off from her career to raise children and is now back at work. She lives in New York with her husband and three sons.

**Cathleen Blood**, a graduate of Yale University, lives in Greenwich CT with her husband and three children. She founded KidsEvents.com and is currently head writer for the website LaughOutLoudMom.com, which feathers a weekly "digital" column with a humorous take on life, love-handles, in-laws, and parenthood.

**Alexandra Bradner** is an assistant professor of philosophy at Denison University, in Granville, Ohio. Before accepting a tenure-track position, she was an instructor at Marshall University, Northwestern University, and the University of Michigan. She is married and has two daughters, who are alternatively smothered and neglected. She received her undergraduate degree from Princeton University and her PhD in philosophy from Northwestern University.

**Majka Burhardt** is the author of *Coffee Story: Ethiopia* (Origin Point Press 2010) and *Vertical Ethiopia: Climbing Toward Possibility in the Horn of Africa* (Shama, 2008). Ms. Burhardt is a frequent lecturer on the intersection of adventure, culture, and environment, and has worked extensively in Africa examining the overlap between the three realms. Executive Producer of the documentary film *Waypoint Namibia* (2009), Burhardt also works as a professional climber and AMGA certified mountain guide. Her work in Africa has been featured on national news programs and radio shows, and in magazines and newspapers throughout the world. Ms. Burhardt holds an MFA in Creative Writing from the Warren Wilson Program for Writers, and received her BA in anthropology from Princeton University. Her website is MajkaBurhardt.com.

**Heather Cabot** spent more than fifteen years as a TV reporter and anchor at networks including ABC News, where she co-anchored *World News Now* and *World News This Morning*. She is the Founder & Editor-in-Chief of TheWellMom.com, a weekly e-zine that empowers moms to better care for themselves in mind, body and spirit. She also serves as the Web Life Editor for Yahoo! As mother of five-year-old twins, she is always on the hunt for tips and inspiration on how to simplify her life.

**Courtney Cook** is a teacher and writer whose essays, reviews and interviews have appeared in *The Washington Post, Salon.com, More* magazine, and American Public Media's *The Story*. Courtney's various roles as mom, teacher, librarian, communications director, step-mom, poet, and free-lance writer have taken her from New Hampshire to Kentucky to Connecticut to Sydney, Australia and back with more than a few interesting bumps along the way. Her essay, *Quartet*, is an excerpt from her memoir-in-progress, *How to Leave a Soldier*. She is a 1993 graduate of Dartmouth College and holds an MFA from the University of Wollongong in New South Wales, Australia.

**Sara Esther Crispe** is the editor and creator of the women's site, TheJewishWoman.org, a project of Chabad.org, where she is a featured writer. Additionally, she is a well-known lecturer and leading speaker of women's issues. Sara Esther recently moved back to the States after living in Jerusalem for eight years where she and her husband were the directors of Torat Chesed: The Institute for Advanced Learning for Jewish Women. She is currently working on a book celebrating gender difference according to Kabbalah. She lives with her husband and four children in Merion, PA.

**Berta Davis**, PhD, is an Assistant Clinical Professor of Psychiatry at UCLA and Co-Director of the couple and sex therapy training program of American Association of Couples and Sex Therapists. She served on the board of directors of the Los Angeles County Psychological Association for over twenty-five years. She is currently in private practice in Encino and Beverly Hills, where she helps individuals and couples cope with the challenging task of balancing career and family.

**Lydia Denworth** is the author of *Toxic Truth: A Scientist, a Doctor, and the Battle Over Lead*. She is a former reporter for *Newsweek* and bureau chief for *People*. Her writing on science, education, and social issues has appeared in *The New York Times, Redbook, Health* and other publications. She has also worked as an adjunct professor of journalism at both Fordham University and Long Island University. She is currently living in Hong Kong with her husband and three sons, but she considers Brooklyn home. You can learn more about Lydia and her work at lydiadenworth.com.

**Deborah Fryer** lives in Boulder, Colorado with her husband, Lon, and her six-year-old Standard Poodle, Lila, whose name in

Sanskrit means "the interconnectedness of everything." She divides her time between filmmaking , freelance writing, teaching yoga, and playing in the mountains. Samples of her video work can be found online at LilaFilms.com.

**Bracha Goetz** serves on the Executive Committee of the national organization, Jewish Board of Advocates for Children, and coordinates a Jewish Big Brothers and Big Sisters Program in Baltimore, Maryland. She is the author of thirteen children's books, including *Remarkable Park, What Do You See in Your Neighborhood?* and *The Invisible Book*. She graduated from Harvard University, attended the Medical College of Virginia, and went on to study at Ohr Someyach Women's Division in Jerusalem.

**Jill Gott-Gleason** "retired" from a career in real estate development and is in her second year as a stay-at-home mom. She writes a fashion and lifestyle blog, GoodLifeForLess.blogspot.com, to relieve boredom and stay connected to the outside world. She graduated from Calvin College in West Michigan and continues to live in the same community with her husband and two children.

**Sara Debbie Gutfreund** lives in Telzstone, Israel with her husband and children. She is a freelance writer and is currently working on her first novel. She holds a BA in English from the University of Pennsylvania and a Masters in Family Therapy from the University of North Texas.

**Barbara G.S. Hagerty** is a native of Charleston, South Carolina, and the mother of four children. Her essays, columns, and poems have appeared in a wide variety of national and regional periodicals. She has written two books, plus a collection of poetry, *The Guest House* (Finishing Line Press, 2009). A member of the Long Table Poets, a biweekly workshop led by Richard Garcia, she currently holds the Fellowship in Poetry from the South Carolina Arts Commission. She has also worked as a photographer, curator, and teacher of poetry and creative nonfiction. She holds an MA in Creative Writing from The Johns Hopkins University.

**Laurie Henneman** is a research scientist and Professor of Biology at the University of Montana Western. She received her PhD in Ecology and Evolutionary Biology from the University of Arizona and her AB from Princeton University. She lives in Montana with her husband and daughter.

**Shelby Hogan** lives in Anaheim, California, with her husband Kevin, their son Theodore, and two beagles. When she's not busy chasing Theo around, she can be found blogging at GenXMomsBlog.com, writing under the name, "The Scrivener." She is currently pursuing an MFA in writing from Vermont College.

**Amy Hudock**, PhD, is a writer, professor, and editor who lives in South Carolina with her family. She is a co-founder of *Literary Mama*, an online literary magazine chosen by Writers Digest as one of the 101 Best Web Sites for Writers (2005 and 2009) and by *Forbes* as one of their 100 Best of the Web (2005). She is also the co-editor of *Literary Mama: Reading for the Maternally Inclined* (Seal Press, 2006) and of the book, *American Women Prose Writers, 1820-1870* (Gale, 2001). Her work has been anthologized in the *Chicken Soup for the Soul* and *Cup of Comfort* series, as well as in *Ask Me About My Divorce, Mama, PhD, Single State of the Union*, and *Mothering a Movement*.

**Nina Misuraca Ignaczak** is an environmental urban planner who dreams of becoming a writer. She has published articles in magazines including the *Michigan Planner, Planning & Zoning News, Orion Magazine, Literary Mama, Babble.com*, as well as her own blog, placeroot.blogspot.com. Nina has a BS in Biology and an MS in Natural Resource Management from the University of Michigan. She resides in the suburbs of Detroit, Michigan, with her husband, son and daughter.

**Joana Jebsen** works full-time in publishing. She is married and lives in a small rural town in Connecticut with her husband and twin daughters, now ten. She majored in Comparative Literature at Princeton and received her MBA from the Wharton School of the University of Pennsylvania.

**Liesl Jurock**, M.Ed., is the author of MamasLog.com, a blog about the joys and contrasts that motherhood offers. Her work has appeared online on The Momoir Project, Hybrid Mom, Women's Post and other mother-related websites. She shares a beautiful life with her hubby, Kevin, and son, Lucas, in British Columbia, Canada.

**Michelle Levine** is a writer, editor and one-time attorney. She currently freelances for New York Family and Patch.com and authors the blog, Cupcakes Are Evil (cupcakes-evil.blogspot.com). Her articles have won awards from the Press Club of Long Island. Michelle is a graduate of the University of Pennsylvania and Brooklyn Law School. She lives in Merrick, New York, with her husband and two children.

**Devorah Lifshutz** is an American writer living in Jerusalem. She writes about her experience raising kids in Israel in her contribution to the anthology, *Call Me Okaasan: Adventures in Multicultural Mothering*.

**Carrie L. Lukas** is the vice president for policy and economics at the Independent Women's Forum and a senior fellow at the Goldwater Institute. She worked previously for U.S. House Representative Christopher Cox as the senior domestic policy analyst for the House Republican Policy Committee and a senior staff member of the Homeland Security Committee. Lukas is the author of *The Politically Incorrect Guide to Women, Sex, and Feminism* (Regnery, 2006). Her commentaries have appeared in numerous newspapers, including *The Washington Post, USA Today, The New York Post, The San Francisco Chronicle* and *The Baltimore Sun*. Lukas appears frequently on television shows such as Fox News Channel's *Your World with Neil Cavuto, Fox Report with Shepard Smith, The O'Reilly Factor, Hannity & Colmes*, CNBC's *Kudlow & Company*, and MSNBC's *Hardball with Chris Matthews*.

**Holly Madden** is an advertising Creative Director and copywriter with over twenty years of experience at some of Boston's top advertising agencies, including Arnold Worldwide and Digitas.

For the past nine years, she has run her own business, specializing in brand positioning, digital and social media marketing, and scriptwriting and marketing for film and video. In her free time, she writes short stories and essays that find the humor in parenthood. Holly has an AB from Harvard College and an MS in Film Production from Boston University. She lives in Massachusetts with her two boys, ages nine and five, and an adopted six-year-old Jack Russell Terrier.

**Darcy Mayers** is a former music industry executive  and the founder/owner of Midnight Feeding, an independent media relations agency. She is raising three noisy kids in a suburb of Boston, where she is a  PTO president, community activist and soccer coach. Darcy co-authored the book, *TO: A True Story in Letters, and* writes the blog, Post Picket Fence. She graduated from Brown University with Honors in 1993.

**Lindsey Mead** is an executive search consultant focused on placing professionals in the alternative investment space. She graduated from Princeton with a BA in English and received an MBA from Harvard Business School. She is also a writer, who publishes daily on ADesignSoVast.com. She lives with her husband and her two children in Cambridge, Massachusetts.

**Susan Morse** is an Associate Professor at the University of California Hastings College of the Law. She was previously an Assistant Research Professor and Teaching Fellow at Santa Clara University School of Law, an associate at the law firms of Wilson Sonsini Goodrich & Rosati and Ropes & Gray, and a clerk on the First Circuit Court of Appeals. She graduated from Princeton University in 1993 and Harvard Law School in 1996. She currently lives in Portola Valley, California, with her husband and three daughters.

**Abi Cotler O'Roarty** teaches photography and design at the Art Institute of California, San Diego. She writes short fiction and personal essays and pens a column on children and motherhood for *The Huffington Post* as well as the *Encinitas Patch Parentspeak* column on Patch.com. In her free time, she can be found raising a preschooler and a baby whose tiny voices penetrate nearly every thought she has.

**Katherine Ozment** is a freelance writer with twenty years of publishing experience, including stints at *Boston* magazine and *National Geographic*. Her musings on the ups and downs of motherhood have been widely published, and her kids are bound to disown her when they're old enough to Google. She lives in Cambridge, Massachusetts, with her husband and three children, and her work can be found at KatherineOzment.com.

**Windi Padia** is the Education Section Manager for a state wildlife agency in Colorado. She writes human interest articles for *Colorado Outdoors Magazine* and blogs at CrazyCopperTop.blogspot.com. Windi graduated from Princeton University in 2000, where she majored in Ecology and Evolutionary Biology.

**Sabrina Parsons** is the CEO of Palo Alto Software and founder of the Web blog, MommyCEO.org. Prior to joining Palo Alto Software, she was a co-founder of Lighting Out Consulting and a Senior Producer at Epinions.com. She is the co-author of a book recently published by Entrepreneur Press, *3 Weeks To Startup*.

**Regan Penaluna** received her PhD in philosophy from Boston University, and she currently teaches at St. John's University in New York. She has written for several publications, including *The Chronicle of Higher Education, Philosophy Now*, and *First Things*. She also blogs for *The Philosophers' Magazine*.

**Katy Read** is a Minneapolis-based writer whose work has appeared in *Salon, More, Brain Child, Real Simple, AARP The Magazine, Working Mother, Parents, River Teeth, Brevity,* the *Minneapolis Star Tribune,* the *Chicago Sun-Times* and many other outstanding publications.

Before becoming a freelance writer, she was a newspaper staff writer, most recently at the *New Orleans Times-Picayune*. She blogs daily at "What I should be doing instead" http://whatishouldbedoinginstead.blogspot.com/

**Sue Repko** is a writer and licensed urban planner. She is the founder of Positively!Pottstown.com, a community blog for her hometown of Pottstown, PA, to assist in its revitalization efforts. She has a BA in psychology from Princeton University and a master's in city and regional planning from Rutgers University. She is currently an MFA candidate in nonfiction at the Bennington Writing Seminars. Her writing has appeared in *The Gettysburg Review, Beloit Fiction Journal, Broken Bridge Review, Bryant Literary Review, New Millennium Writings, flashquake, the Princeton Alumni Weekly*, and *The Literary Traveler*. She lives in central New Jersey with her husband of twenty-five years and their two teenage sons.

**Amy Schneider** worked as a business analyst for The Advisory Board Company in Washington, DC, and as a management consultant for Diamond Technology Partners, now part of PriceWaterhouseCoopers. Currently, she stays at home with her two children in Northern New Jersey, where she spends her time organizing kids' activities for the local newcomers group and driving her children all over town. She has a degree from Princeton University in East Asian Studies and an MBA from MIT.

**Jessica Scott** spent nearly twelve years in the U.S. Army as a senior NCO before she commissioned as an officer in 2007. She has over fourteen years as both officer and enlisted, and has lived in Korea, Germany, and most recently, Fort Hood, Texas. She is one half of a dual military couple and is the mother to two young daughters. She deployed in 2009 with the First Cavalry Division, where she wrote regularly from Iraq about her experiences as a deployed mom and a woman at war, and about leadership during combat operations. Her work has been featured on *The New York Times* "At War" blog. She holds a BA in Cultural Studies and an MS in Telecommunications Management.

**Katherine Shaver** is a staff writer for *The Washington Post*, where she has covered crime, education, government, development and transportation since 1997. She previously wrote about criminal justice issues for the *St. Petersburg Times* and covered Congress for newspapers in California and Florida. She has been grateful to work part-time since her first child was born. She lives in the Washington, DC area with her husband and two children. She is a graduate of Princeton University.

**Alaina Sheer** writes about life, love and motherhood on her blog, MsSingleMama.com. A single mother to her son Benjamin, Alaina is also the Chief Digital Strategist of Cement Marketing, a company she created, in large part, to have more freedom as a working mother. She has been quoted in The Guardian, The Chicago Tribune, WBNS-10 TV, Columbus Monthly and on CNN.com.

**Karen Sibert, MD** is an anesthesiologist in private practice in Los Angeles, California. She received an AB degree in English from Princeton University, graduating in 1974, and attended medical school at Baylor College of Medicine in Houston, Texas. She is the mother of four – Arden, Alexandra (who died in infancy), Thomas, and Ariel – and is married to Steven M. Haddy, MD, who practices cardiac anesthesiology at the University of Southern California. In what spare time she has, she reads novels, walks her dog, and studies Arabic.

**Joan-Dianne Smith** is a clinical social worker and psychotherapist in private practice in Winnipeg, Canada. She attended Wilfrid Laurier University in Ontario and Smith College in Massachusetts. She has published her writing in *The Globe and Mail, The Dalhousie Review, Cahoots Magazine*, and in the recent anthology, *Christmas Chaos: twenty-five original stories of Christmas gone awry* by Prairie Dog Publishing. She is married with three children.

**Ashley Stone** is a stay-at-home mom, a work-at-home mom, and a blogger (OurFamilyStone.org) on the side. She has two beautiful little girls who fill her life with love, joy, and exhaustion.

**Shannon Hyland-Tassava** is a writer, clinical psychologist, and mom to two daughters. She lives in a Midwest college town with her family, and chronicles the chaos and delight of modern motherhood on her blog, MamaInWonderland.blogspot.com. Shannon has written for a variety of print and Web-based publications, including *Motherwords* magazine, *Macalester Today* magazine, BlogHer, The Mothers Movement Online, WorkitMom.com, and the anthology *P.S. What I Didn't Say: Unsent Letters to Our Female Friends*. She writes a health and wellness column for her local newspaper, and is currently working on a nonfiction book about stay-at-home motherhood.

**Tracy Thompson** is a professional journalist and author who lives in the Washington, DC, suburbs with her husband and two daughters. She worked for *The Washington Post* and *The Atlanta Constitution*, where her series "Rural Justice" was selected as a finalist for the 1988 Pulitzer Prize in Investigative Reporting. She has authored two books, *The Beast* (Plume, 1996) and *The Ghost in the House: Motherhood, Raising Children and Struggling with Depression* (HarperCollins, 2006). Her stories have also been included in two anthologies, *The Healing Circle* (Plume, 1998) and *Out of Her Mind: Women Writing on Madness* (2000). She currently chronicles her experience with motherhood and depression on her blog, MaternallyChallenged.typepad.com.

**Kim Todd** is the author of *Chrysalis, Maria Sibylla Merian and the Secrets of Metamorphosis* (Harcourt, 2007) and *Tinkering with Eden, a Natural History of Exotics in America* (W.W. Norton, 2001). She has taught environmental and nature writing at the University of Montana, the University of California at Santa Cruz, and the Environmental Writers Institute. She currently teaches at Penn State, The Behrend College, and is a senior fellow with the Environmental Leadership Program. Kim has an MFA in creative nonfiction and an MS in environmental studies, both from the University of Montana, and a BA in English from Yale.

**Jennifer Ulveling**, JD/MBA, is an attorney and psychotherapy intern. In addition, she is a mother, a wife, a short-order chef, an arts director, and a general manager of all things domestic. She resides in Oakland, California, with her husband, her two children and the growing realization that she can't do it all.

**Kezia Willingham** is a former high-school dropout, single mother, and welfare recipient, who has a bachelor's degree from Oregon State University and a master's in social work from the University of Washington. She resides in Seattle, where she works for the Head Start program and is an advocate for immigration reform. She credits the memoirs of other mothers as guiding lights in time of darkness. She is married with three children.

# ABOUT THE AUTHOR/EDITOR

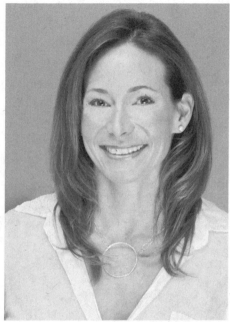

Courtesy of Frank Fennema

**Samantha Parent Walravens** is an award-winning journalist, writer and mother of four children. She was an editor for *PC World* magazine before leaving journalism to chase the "Internet dream" in the mid-1990s. She has since returned to her true passion, writing, and has published articles on topics including politics, business, lifestyle and women's issues. Samantha is a Phi Beta Kappa graduate of Princeton University and has a Master's in Literature and Women's Studies from the University of Virginia. *Torn: True Stories of Kids, Career & the Conflict of Modern Motherhood* is her first book. For more information, visit her website: www.samanthawalravens.com.